"Dr Kanji has produced a superb book on lower back pain. He has clearly explained what causes lower back pain, the investigations that are useful and the solutions to reduce lower back pain. I have no doubt this will be a number one selling lower back pain book. The illustrations are amazing. Well donc."

Vijay Vallabh, Physiotherapist/Director Proactive Rehab Ltd

"I recommend this book to all my patients to ensure they understand their lower back pain and can self-manage their pain. The book is very easy to read and explains what the various radiological tests show with real images throughout thc book. Three years in the writing, this has been worth waiting for. The finished product is superb."

Brett Bulkeley, Chiropractor

"This is the book I have been waiting for to recommend to all my patients with lower back pain. A simple book that is easy to read."

Dr Stu Thomson, Sports Doctor

"Dr Kanji has treated many of my patients for lower back pain, his straight-foward simple approach, is outlined in this exemplary book which should help the many people around the world who suffer from lower back pain."

Dr Ian Coutts, Consultant Physician

Fix Your Back

DR GIRESH KANJI

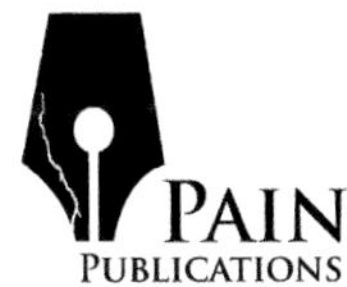

First published in June 2013 by Pain Publications,
Level 2, 354 Lambton Quay, Wellington, New Zealand
Second edition, November 2013

National Library of New Zealand Cataloguing-in-Publication Data
Kanji, Giresh, 1966-
Fix Your Back
author; Giresh Kanji ; editor Rachel Page.
Includes bibliographical references.
ISBN 978-0-473-26735-3
1. Backache—Popular works. 2. Backache—Treatment—Popular works. I. Page, Rachel Audrey. II. Title.
617.564—dc 23

Editor: Associate Professor Rachel Page
Cover design: Preehya Patel
Illustrator: Preehya Patel
Printed by Printlink, Wellington, New Zealand

www.painpublications.com

About the author

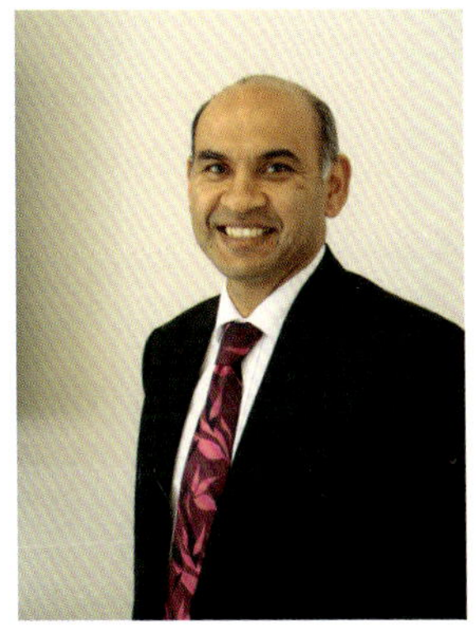

Dr Giresh Kanji was born in Wellington, New Zealand, and educated at Wellington College, Otago Medical School and Massey University. He has worked as a medical doctor since 1990 and qualified as a Musculoskeletal Pain Specialist in 2002, focusing on chronic pain disorders. He finished a PhD investigating chronic pain in 2013. Dr Kanji is the Chairperson of the New Zealand Pain Foundation set up to perform research on mental and physical pain disorders. Giresh lives in Wellington with his wife and three children.

Contents

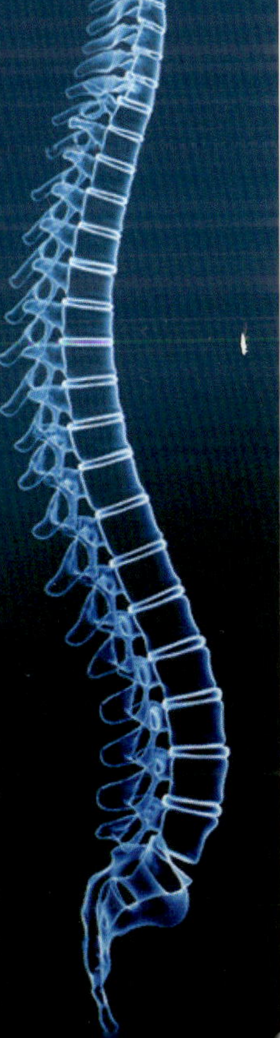

INTRODUCTION **1**
Solving the puzzle of pain 1

1 LOWER BACK PAIN **3**

2 HOW DO WE EXPERIENCE PAIN? **9**
What is pain? 10
Referred pain 13

3 WHAT CAUSES LOWER BACK PAIN? **17**
The muscles of the lower back 19
The ligaments and tendons 21
The disc 22
The facet joint 34
Variations of the spine 37
The hip 37
The sacro-iliac joint 42

4 INVESTIGATING LOWER BACK PAIN **47**
X-ray 49
MRI scan 51
CT scan 53
Bone scan 53

5 THE EIGHT GOLDEN RULES FOR MANAGING LOWER BACK PAIN **55**
Avoid heavy lifting 56
Maintain the lower back curve 56
Maintain good sitting posture 59
Maintain good bending posture 62
Lift with good technique 64
Try inversion therapy 65
Ensure good sleeping posture 69

Maintain core strength 71

6 TREATING LOWER BACK PAIN 77
Medications 79
Manual therapy 82
Massage 82
Mobilisation 82
Manipulation 83
Needle therapies for lower back pain 83
Acupuncture 84
Injections 84
Surgery for lower back pain 86
Discectomy 86
Fusion 87
Disc replacement 88

7 CHRONIC LOWER BACK PAIN 91
The adrenaline nightmare 92
The alcohol hangover 92
The fight/flight response 94
Depleting stress chemicals 95
Sleep disturbance and fatigue 97
Conclusion 100

GLOSSARY 101
REFERENCES 105
INDEX 106
ACKNOWLEDGEMENTS 108

Introduction

I started working full time in pain medicine over ten years ago and recall going to work with a feeling of dread. What was I going to do to help these patients? Prescribe medication that never seemed to cure the suffering and often caused side effects? I was no longer happy prescribing medications without trying to understand the cause of people's pain. I decided to investigate why people developed pain and how to reduce it.

After years of treating chronic pain patients, I noticed that pain spreads and intensifies with time, making it difficult to diagnose its source. Often the patient's pain may no longer be at the site of injury and the diagnosis becomes blurred for both the patient and the health professional.

Chronic lower back pain is a significant worldwide medical puzzle with reportedly no cause found in up to 85% of cases[1]. So what do you do when you cannot find the cause and treat pain? Call in the psychologist and psychiatrist to help people cope with their symptoms? I feel that the medical profession has failed these patients. Many patients do not understand why they are seeking psychological help, often feeling that the doctor thinks the problem is in their head! After seeing numerous specialists without any answers, a patient may believe this to be true.

My journey into examining the chronic pain puzzle started in earnest back in July 2005. I was researching a presentation on referred pain for the New Zealand Association of Musculoskeletal Medicine conference in Dunedin, New Zealand. I became curious about where people's pain comes from, how it spreads and amplifies, and why almost everyone with chronic pain develops problems such as insomnia, anxiety, depression and mental irritability.

I became fascinated and spent several years examining scientific literature to try and solve the puzzle of pain. I read books on biochemistry, neurophysiology, neurology, and the sympathetic nervous system (stress nervous system) and made countless computer searches on various topics. I would wake between four and five a.m. and read and write for several hours before work. This habit remained for many years as the puzzle of pain started unfolding. During this time I completed two business degrees and read many books on critical thinking. The biggest lesson I learned was to keep asking why until a satisfactory answer is found, otherwise you only get half-truths and half-cures.

My journey culminated in spending five years working towards a PhD thesis. I created a model to explain why pain amplifies and spreads throughout the body after examining over 600 scientific papers and dozens of books.

I wanted to find the cause of people's pain and reduce their pain scores to zero (zero being no pain, ten being the worst pain imaginable). If a patient's pain could not be eliminated I hoped to find its cause, as the most frustrating thing for patients is not knowing what is causing their pain. Furthermore, if the source of pain is known, then treatment can be targeted at the problem. If no treatment is available, then time and money need not be wasted on therapy that may not help.

This book describes what structures in the lower back cause pain, how pain is transmitted, and what can be done about it. I hope to reach people who are suffering and provide some explanation of their symptoms, outline investigations that can be performed, and describe possible treatment options.

My thanks go out to all the patients who have allowed their stories to appear in this book. All names have been changed so patients cannot be identified.

1 LOWER BACK PAIN

Lower back pain

Lower back pain can be thought of as part of the human condition. Just like catching the flu, it is hard to avoid and makes you feel miserable. In fact, it affects nearly everyone at some time in their lives[2]. Between 60 and 70 percent of people will improve from an initial episode of lower back pain within six weeks. Only two to five percent of people will seek treatment for their lower back pain and may require time off work. For a third of people the pain lasts up to seven weeks, with many people having three to four recurrences per year. A small proportion of people experience daily pain for many years.

In my practice I have noticed that people who have had an injury often improve and then have episodes of lower back pain whenever they perform heavy lifting, bending or strenuous activities, even several decades after their initial injury. These episodes of pain often result from the irritation of the initial injured structure.

People with chronic lower back pain often endure nights of broken sleep, and feel tired, irritable, anxious and depressed. The suffering is worse when they have no explanation for their pain. They worry about what is wrong with them, what the future holds and whether they will ever get better. They try every treatment, vitamin or mineral known to mankind only to find themselves disappointed.

While lower back pain is a burden to individuals, it is also a significant and costly problem in Western societies. Each year the number of people who suffer lower back pain and cannot work increases. The workers' compensation available in the West has placed a financial burden on the economy. However the money received by those on workers' compensation rarely makes up for the immense suffering they endure.

A logical approach to treating lower back pain is to exclude structures that can cause pain one at a time, initially using simple treatments and progressing to more invasive treatments. Any structure with a nerve supply is capable of causing pain. Ligaments, tendons, muscles, bones, discs and joints are all possible sources of pain with the disc being the most common source of pain.

For practical purposes, the tissues that cause pain are best separated into soft tissues (ligaments, muscles, tendons) and hard tissues (bones, facet joints and discs). If someone gets 100 percent relief of their pain from treatment to the soft tissues of the lower back, then it would seem reasonable to conclude that their pain was caused by soft tissues. Those improving by 50 percent may have had some pain caused by their soft tissues, however other deeper structures are also likely to be contributing to their pain.

The structures of the lower back are only part of the story. They cannot cause pain without the pathways that detect and transmit pain. The pain pathways include sensors (pressure, stretch, chemical and pain), pain switches and nerves. The pain pathways conduct tiny electrical signals that result in the experience of pain. To understand lower back pain it is imperative to understand how pain is transmitted through the body as described in Chapter 2.

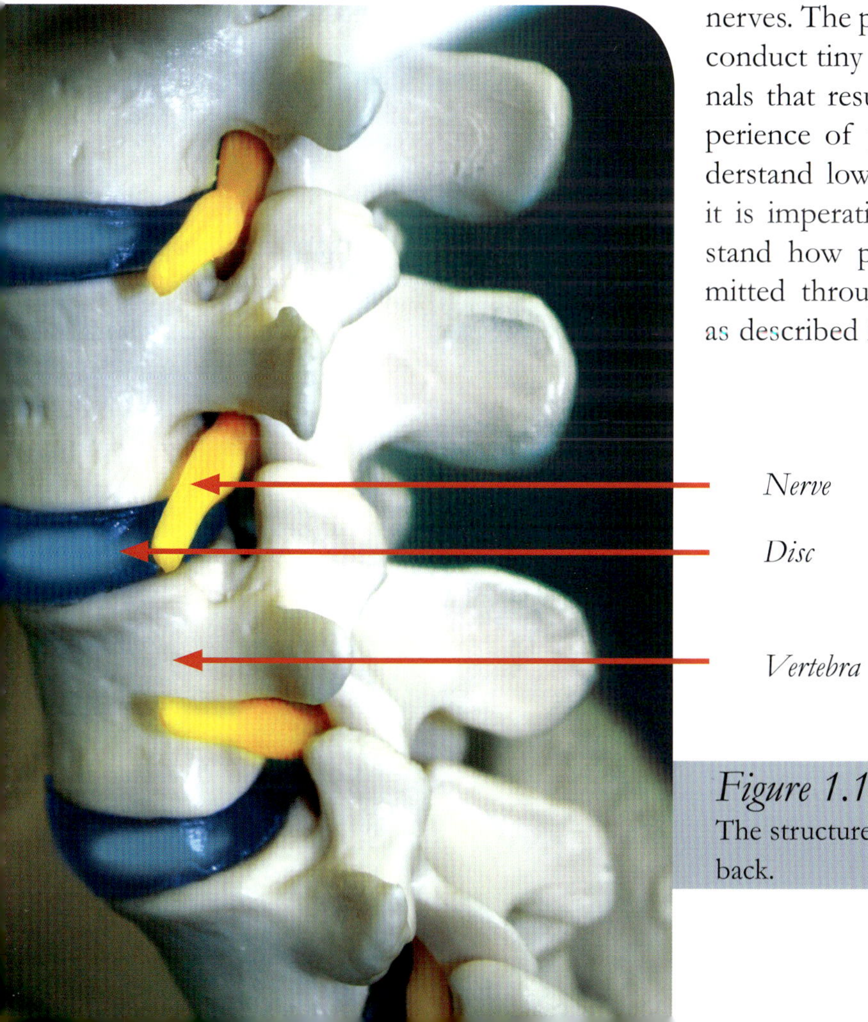

Nerve

Disc

Vertebra

Figure 1.1
The structures of the lower back.

CASE STUDY: *John*

John's lower back pain started 16 years before he presented, when he slipped and landed on his back while working as a welder. Despite seeing several health professionals including spine specialists and undergoing many rehabilitation programmes, he had found no relief from his pain and suffering. John had just turned 63 years old and had been advised by his insurance company that his lower back pain was due to the ageing process. He was about to lose his weekly insurance payments.

John could not live on his own as he had difficulty standing, sitting and walking for any distance. He could not even stand in the queue at the bank or supermarket without his pain increasing. His daughter had been his live-in caregiver for the previous ten years, performing all the housework and cooking duties.

I saw John for his lower back pain and after three treatments of saline injections into the lower back muscles and ligaments his lower back pain improved substantially. He was able to walk freely without restriction, perform his own housework and cooking and even started working in a voluntary job for a local charity shop six days a week. His daughter left home as she was no longer required to care for him.

John took the insurance company to court and contested the decision that his pain was due to the ageing process. This decision seemed illogical as he was now pain-free and able to participate in all activities without taking any tablets. He also slept well and was back to his old self. He won his day in court and received a payout from the insurance company.

Figure 1.2 shows John's MRI scan. As you can see, the lowest disc has lost fluid and narrowed slightly compared to the above discs. The disc may have been John's initial source of pain, however his case illustrates that the soft tissues were responsible for most of his ongoing pain.

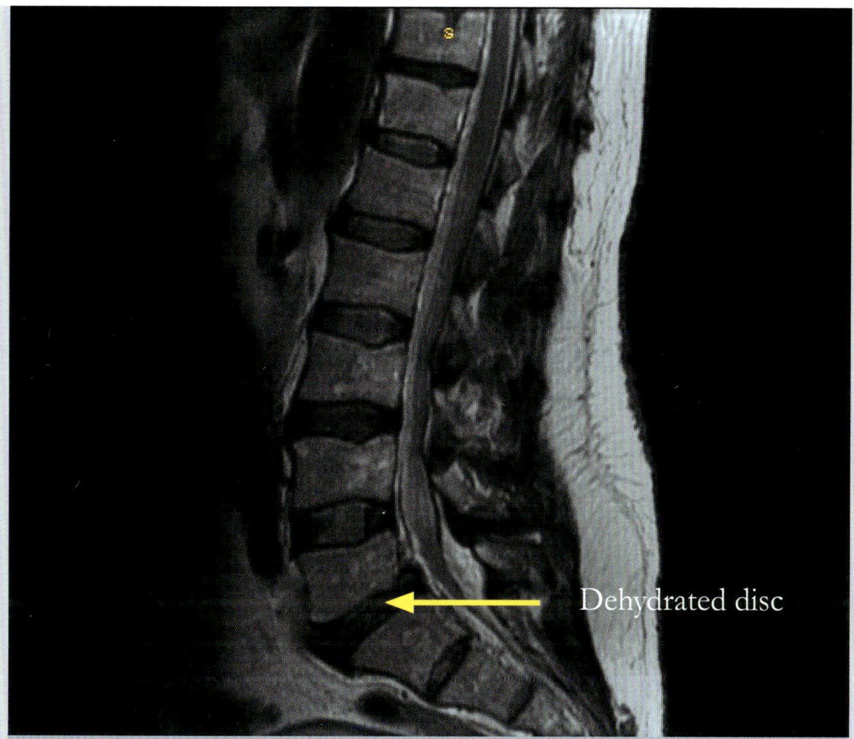

Figure 1.2 John's MRI scan shows good disc heights with dehydration of the lowest lumbar spine disc.

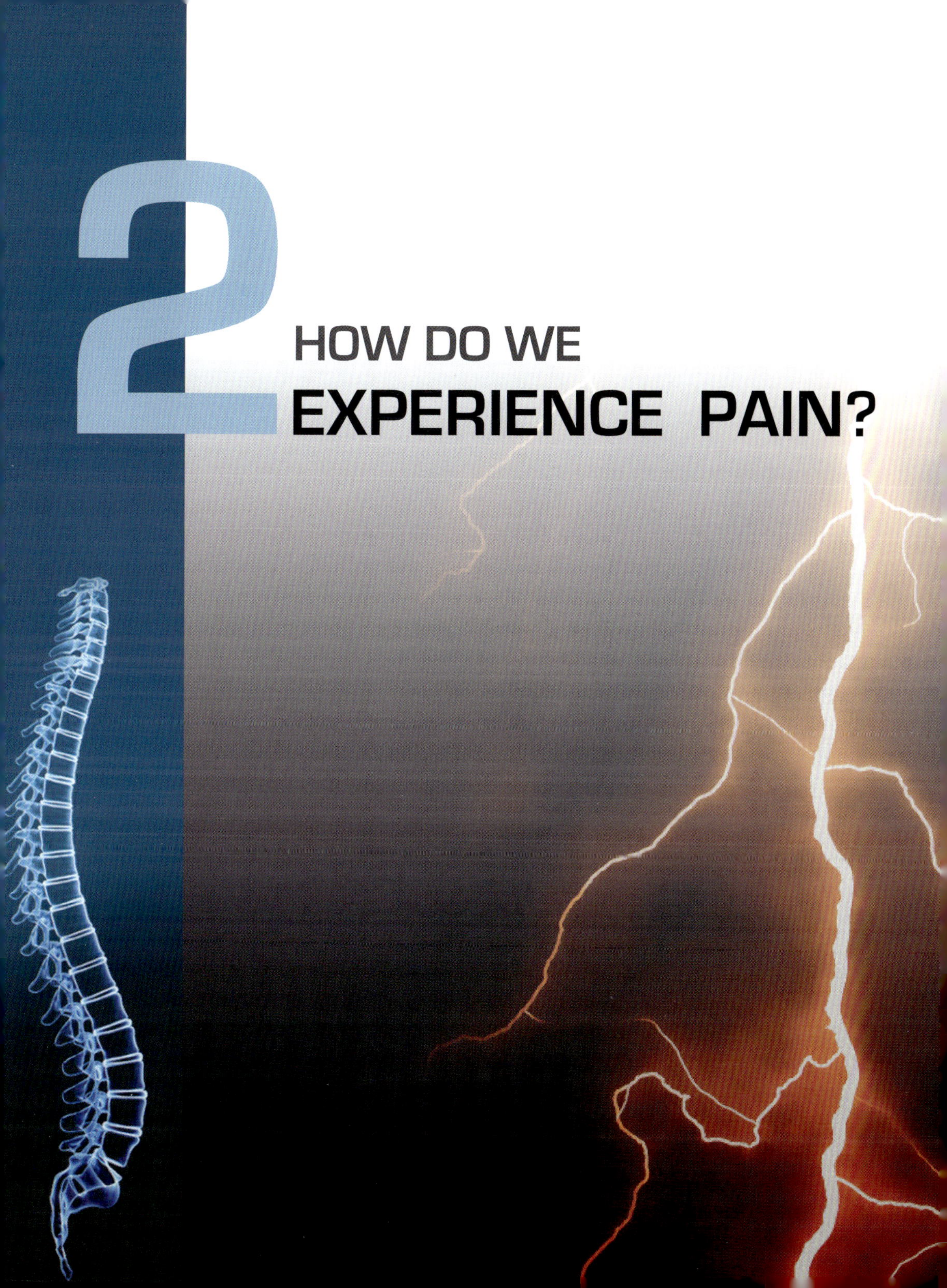

2 HOW DO WE EXPERIENCE PAIN?

What is pain?

Pain is defined as an unpleasant sensory and emotional experience. But how is it produced and how does the brain know that a part of the body has been injured? Receptors are present in the skin, muscles, joints, ligaments, tendons and discs, and they detect pressure, stretch, chemicals, heat and pain. Once a receptor is activated, an electrical spark is generated that is transmitted along nerves to the brain *(Figure 2.1)* like electricity travelling through copper wires. Without electricity conduction, there is no pain.

So essentially, when you feel a pinprick, the skin damage is sensed by pain and pressure receptors, creating an electrical spark that travels through switches in the spinal cord and brain and is interpreted as pain. The brain forms a picture of the site of pain and its intensity, and even sends messages to the emotional parts of the brain.

Sometimes pressure in the joints and the discs of the lower back can cause pain because pressure creates electrical sparks that can be experienced as pain. Hence if you have knee pain, it is often less on sitting than after a long walk.

The level of pain experienced may vary for different individuals depending on several factors. Firstly, the greater the amount of damage, the greater the pain experienced because more receptors are creating electrical sparks. Secondly, when pain is present for months or years the intensity can increase and thirdly, the sensitivity of your pain pathways sets the level of pain experienced.

So what determines the sensitivity of your pain pathways? Your sensitivity to pain is often hereditary and can be increased by stress chemicals. Migraine is a condition which predisposes a person to amplify sensations of sound, light, pain, touch and smell. People who experience migraine have an increased sensitivity to pain because the electrical channels that open to create electricity in the brain open more easily. This increases the electricity

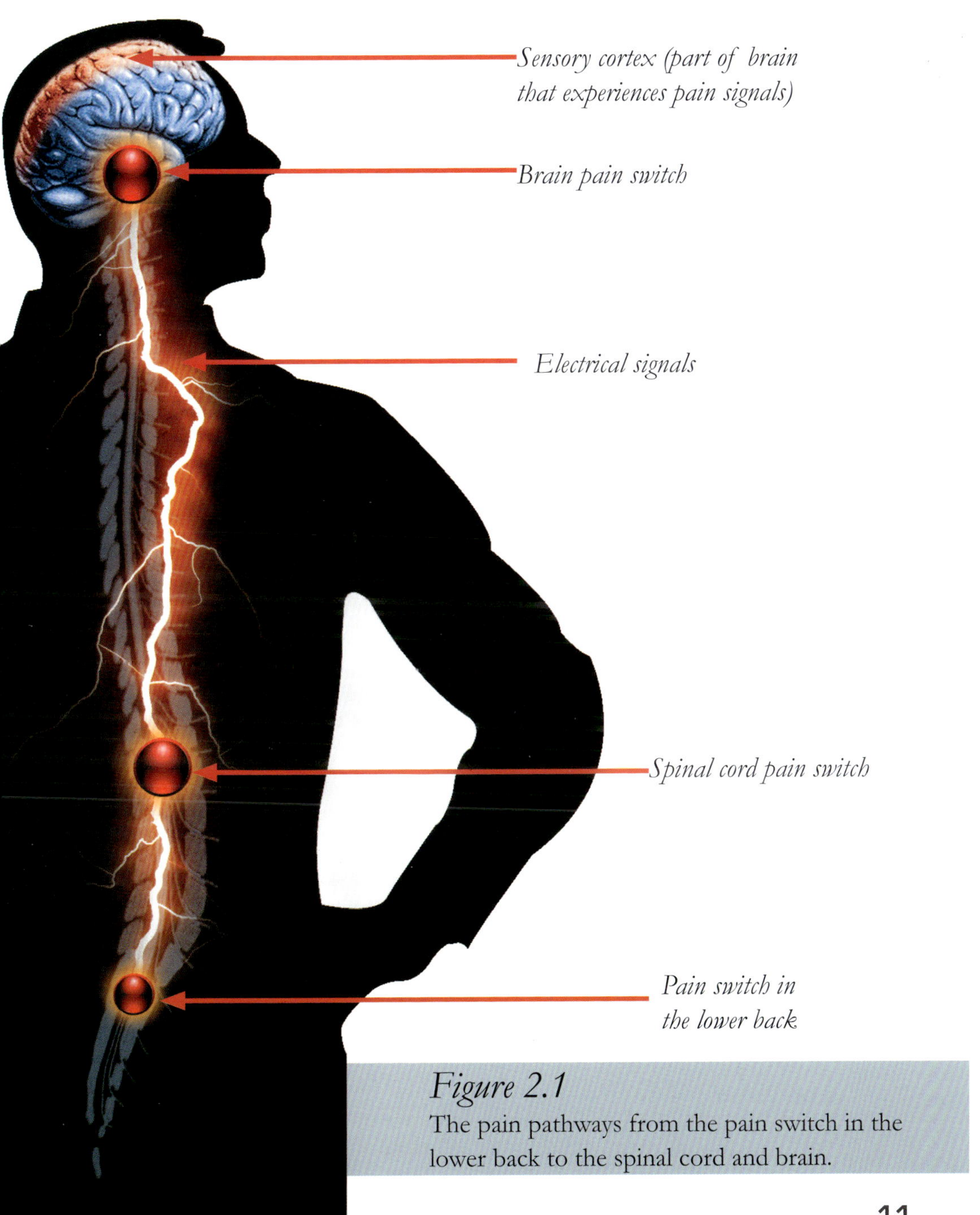

Figure 2.1
The pain pathways from the pain switch in the lower back to the spinal cord and brain.

conducted to the brain, therefore during migraine attacks innocuous sensations such as light and sound become uncomfortable, hence lying in a dark, quiet room is preferred.

For any given injury in the lower back, a person who experiences migraine will experience more intense pain. Moreover, a migraine sufferer who is under stress will experience even more pain. The stress chemicals can in fact activate the migraine gene, explaining why migraine sufferers will experience frequent episodes of migraine headache when under stress and then have minimal symptoms for several months.

Why does your pain become worse when you get stressed? The answer to this question lies in the fact that stress chemicals can attach to your pain pathways and increase electricity, increasing the intensity of pain. Unfortunately, pain itself can cause the body to release stress chemicals leading to a vicious cycle whereby pain creates stress chemicals which amplify pain leading to an ever worsening experience of pain for the patient.

There are two other problems that can arise from the release of stress chemicals: the development of stress-related illnesses, such as insomnia, anxiety and depression; and the spread of pain to other parts of the body, known as referred pain. Once pain has spread there is no simple explanation for the cause of patients' symptoms. If pain is experienced only in the lower back then doctors can easily deduce that a structure in the lower back is likely to be the source of that pain. If pain spreads into the buttock, leg, upper back or throughout the body, then diagnosing the problem is more difficult.

Another important question is what determines which activities will hurt and which activities will be pain-free? For lower back pain, activities that increase pressure on damaged structures such as the discs will be painful. Lifting, bending forward, sneezing or coughing all increase pressure in the disc and can create pain. Sometimes pressure can build up over time, such as when sitting for long periods, increasing pain. Often the pain is worse when sitting on a hard wooden chair compared to a soft padded chair because pressure is absorbed by the soft surface.

In summary, pain is experienced when a receptor detects an injury to a body part and creates an electrical spark that is transmitted to the brain to create the sensation of pain. Switches in the spinal cord and brain are capable of amplifying or diminishing pain. The amount of pain experienced depends on the extent of the damage to the body, the pressure placed on the injured structure, the body's pain sensitivity and the level of stress chemicals in the body.

Referred pain

Referred pain is experienced at a site other than the original site of pain[3]. People who experience lower back pain may also experience pain in their buttocks and legs due to two separate reasons. First, the brain may perceive the pain to be arising from the leg, when it is in fact arising from the lower back (referred pain). There is no damage to the leg even though pain is experienced in the leg.

As the intensity of pain increases, referred pain spreads further. As lower back pain increases pain may spread to the buttock and then down into the leg, often reaching the foot, as shown in *Figure 2.2*. However, once lower back pain improves, the pain recedes into the lower back.

Another reason you can develop leg symptoms from the lower back is because long nerves that start in the lower back travel to the lower leg and foot. These nerves can be irritated in the lower back when they are compressed by a prolapsed disc *(Figure 2.3)* resulting in symptoms of sharp shooting pain, pins and needles, and numbness and tingling in the leg, often to the level of the foot. Weakness can also develop as the nerve is instrumental in maintaing power to the muscles of the leg. Symptoms from nerve irritation are often experienced in one leg but can be experienced in both legs, depending on the size and spread of the disc prolapse.

Nerve compression and referred pain spread pain beyond the soure of the patients' symptoms. Knowing what is the source of the pain is essential to managing and alleviating pain. Chapter 3 examines the various sources of lower back pain.

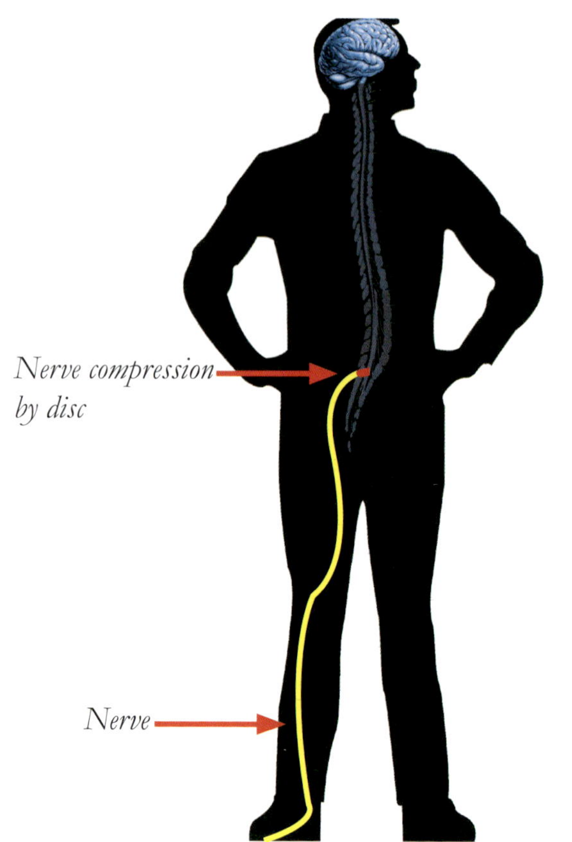

Figure 2.2
The nerves that exit the lower back travel down the leg and into the foot. When they are compressed or irritated they can cause pain and pins and needles down the leg. Numbness and weakness in the leg may also develop.

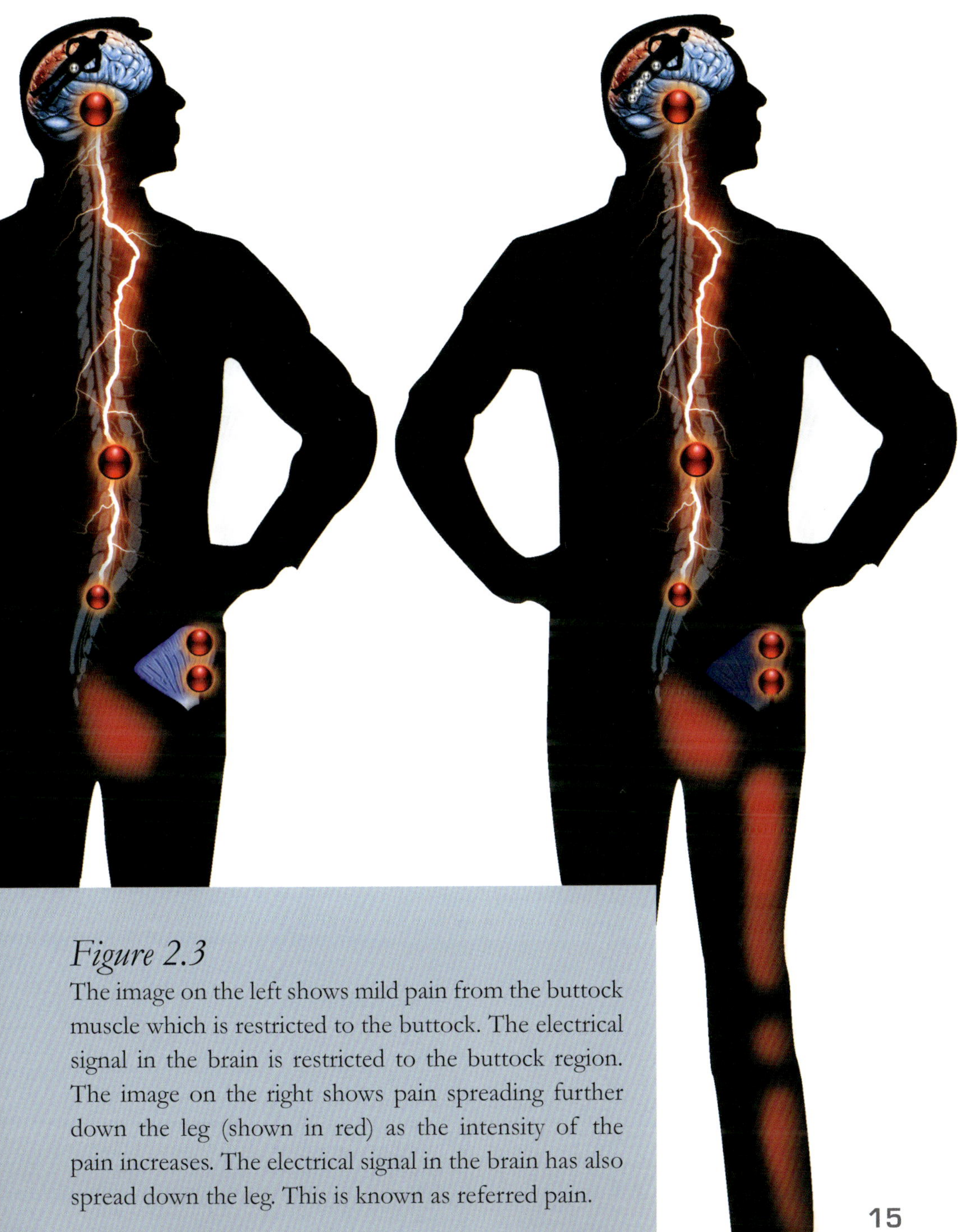

Figure 2.3

The image on the left shows mild pain from the buttock muscle which is restricted to the buttock. The electrical signal in the brain is restricted to the buttock region. The image on the right shows pain spreading further down the leg (shown in red) as the intensity of the pain increases. The electrical signal in the brain has also spread down the leg. This is known as referred pain.

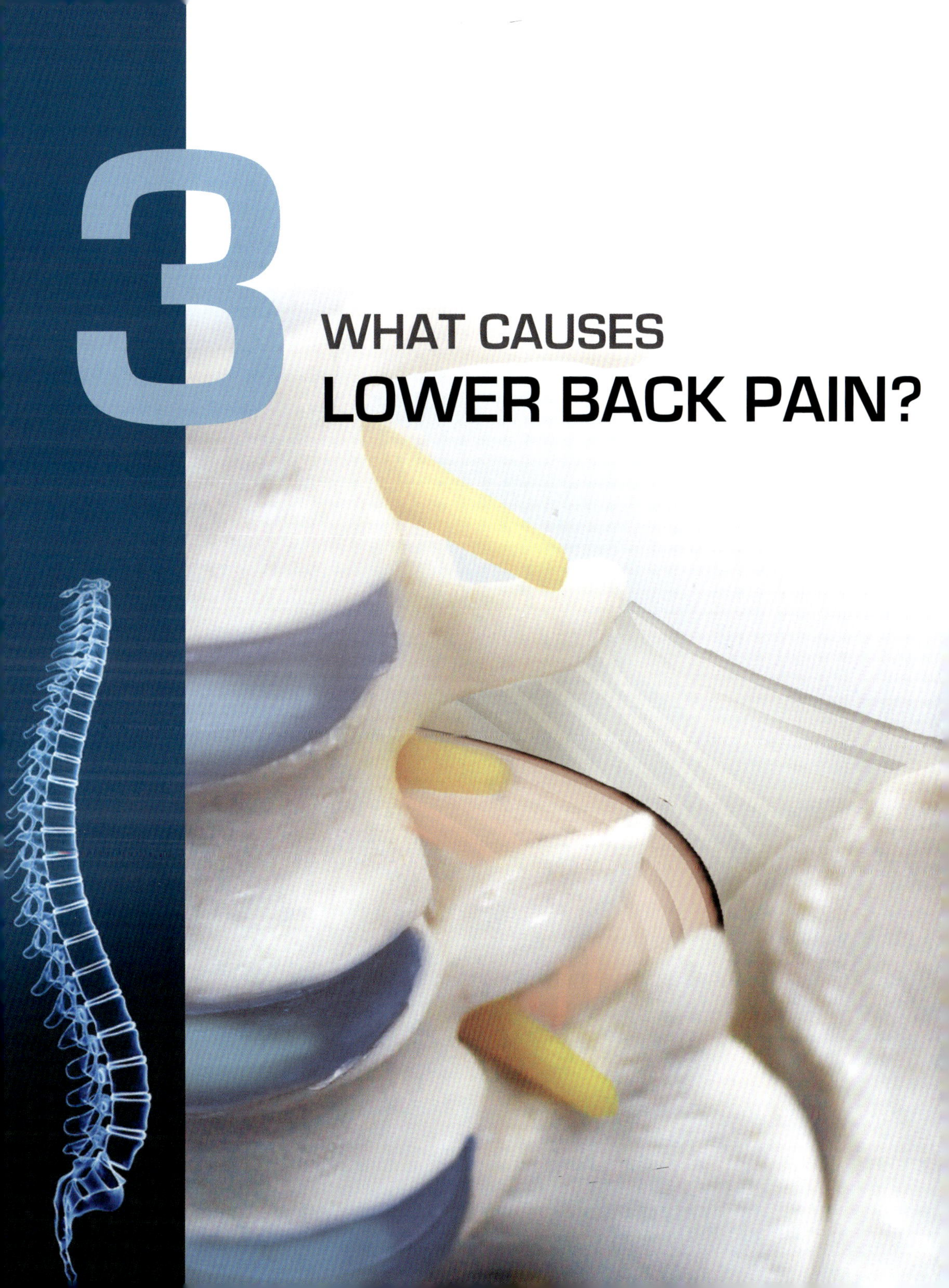

3 WHAT CAUSES LOWER BACK PAIN?

The spinal column consists of 24 bones called vertebrae with discs in between that act as shock absorbers and allow flexibility of the spine. The lower back (lumbar spine) consists of five vertebrae that are commonly called L1 to L5 (*Figure 3.1*). There are pairs of joints at the back of the spine that prevent excessive movement of the lower back called the facet joints. There are also several ligaments in front of and behind the spine. Discs are the most common source of pain in the lower back.

As previously stated, any structure with a nerve supply in the lower back is capable of causing pain, including the muscles, ligaments, tendons, discs, joints and bones.

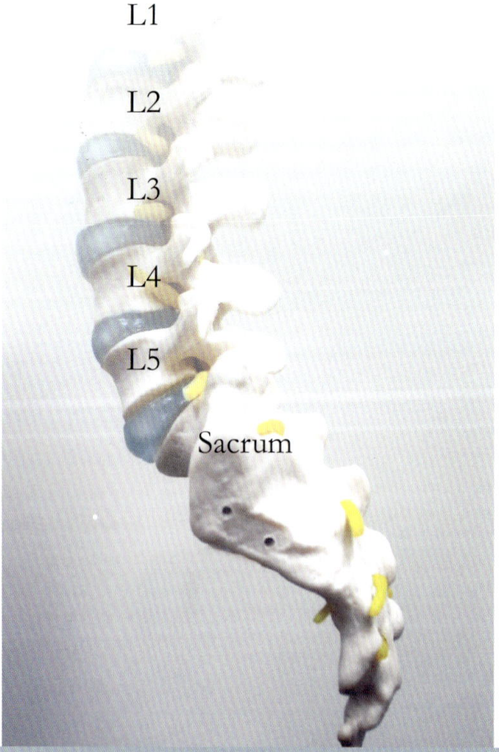

Figure 3.1

The levels of the lower back showing the discs and vertebrae.

CASE STUDY: *Sue*

Sue had experienced low back and buttock pain, mostly on the left side, for 13 years prior to visiting my clinic. Seven years previous to our meeting, while Sue was giving birth, this pain became worse. The pain was better on standing and worse on sitting. Sitting in a car or on a sofa aggravated her pain. Lying down also increased her pain and as a result her sleep was disturbed every night. She often woke during the night and walked around her house in an attempt to alleviate her discomfort.

When I examined Sue, the only positive finding was tenderness over the muscles and ligaments on the left side of her lower back. These were injected with saline and, on her review a few weeks later she had a 70 percent reduction in symptoms. She was sleeping better, her energy had returned and she was able to perform more activities without pain. Although all of her pain had not resolved, a portion of her pain was likely to be stemming from the muscles and ligaments.

When I reviewed Sue several months later, her improvement had continued. She was sleeping well, was able to perform her normal activities and no longer required painkillers.

The muscles of the lower back

The muscles surrounding the lower back and buttock can cause back pain and refer pain into the leg. The patterns of referred pain from many of the lower back muscles have been well-researched. Some of these patterns are shown in *Figures 3.2 to 3.4*.

Figure 3.2
The red shows the referred pain pattern of the gluteus maximus muscle.

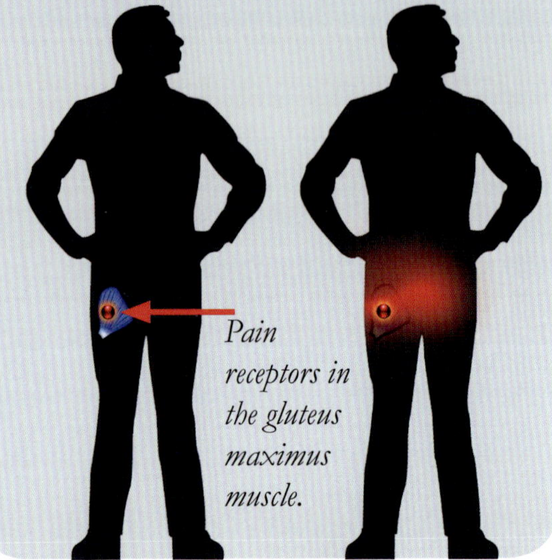

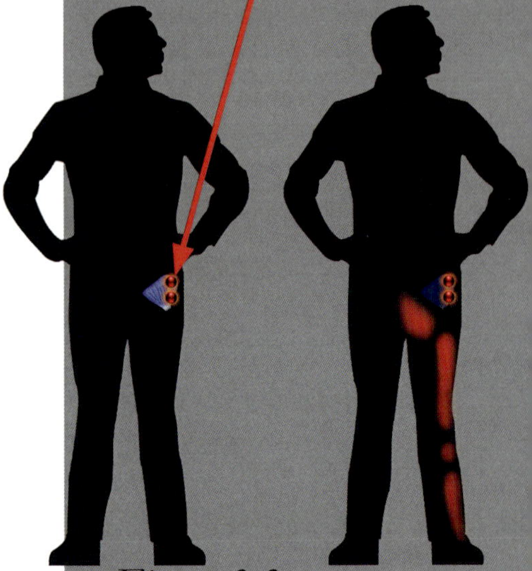

Pain receptors in the gluteus minimus muscle.

Figure 3.3
The red shows the referred pain pattern of the gluteus minimus muscle.

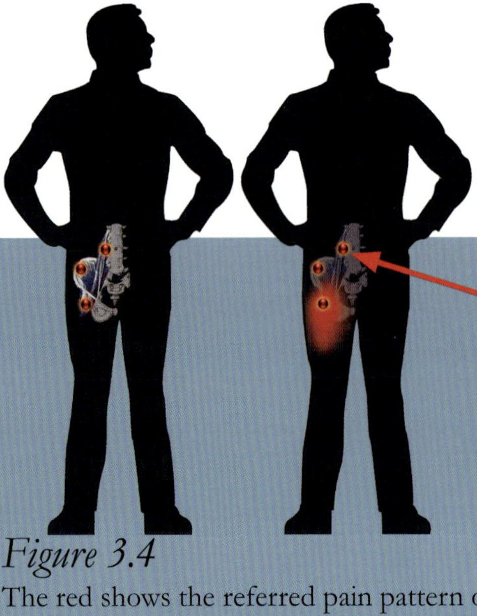

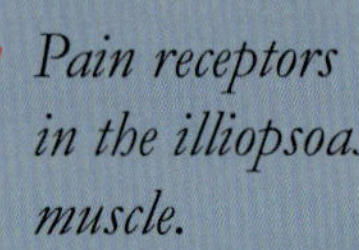

Figure 3.4
The red shows the referred pain pattern of the illiopsoas muscle.

The ligaments and tendons

Ligaments are leather-strap-like structures that hold two bones together, while tendons attach a muscle to bone. There are several tendons and ligaments surrounding the lower back that can cause lower back pain and refer pain into the buttock and leg, as shown in *Figure 3.5*. There is no definitive test to diagnose tendon or ligament pain but examination may reveal tenderness. If treatment aimed at the tendons or ligaments successfully reduces pain, then it can be assumed that these structures were contributing to the pain. Treatment of ligaments may include manual therapy such as friction massage, electrical therapies or injections. Injection solutions can include steroids, prolotherapy or saline.

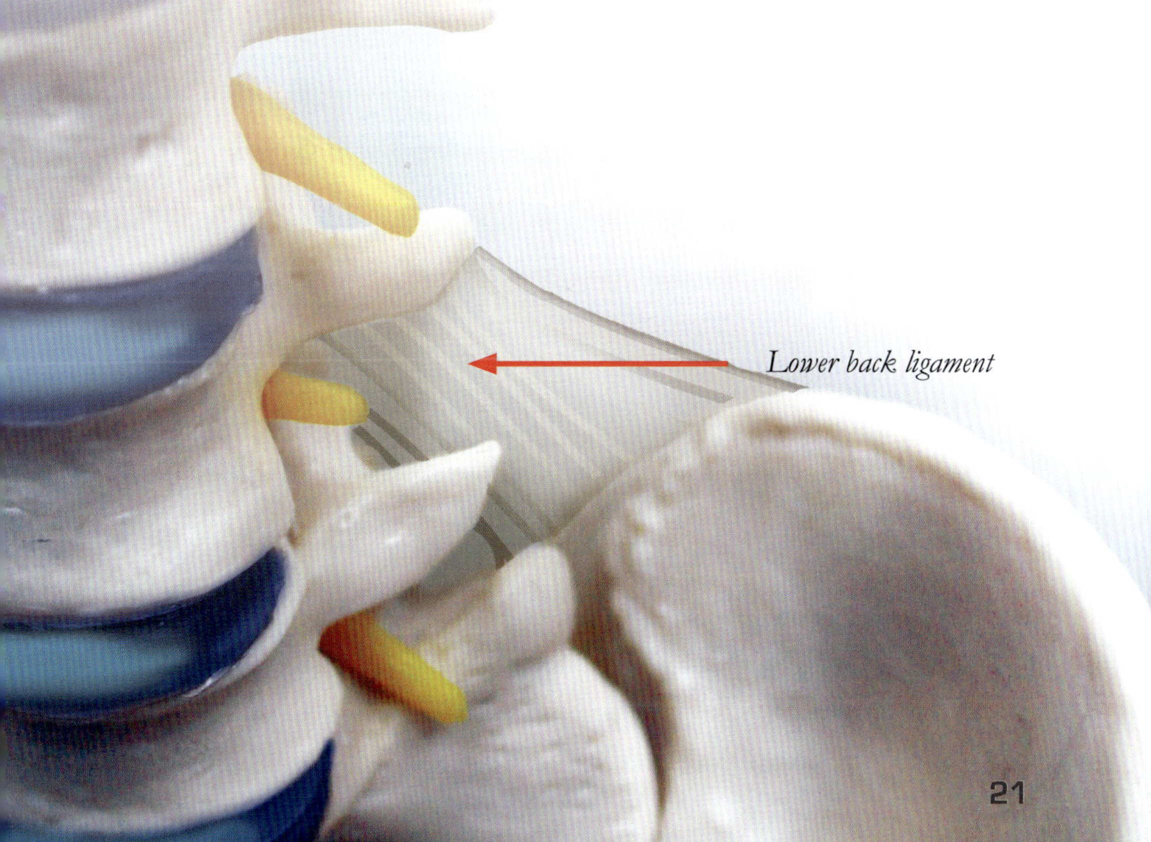

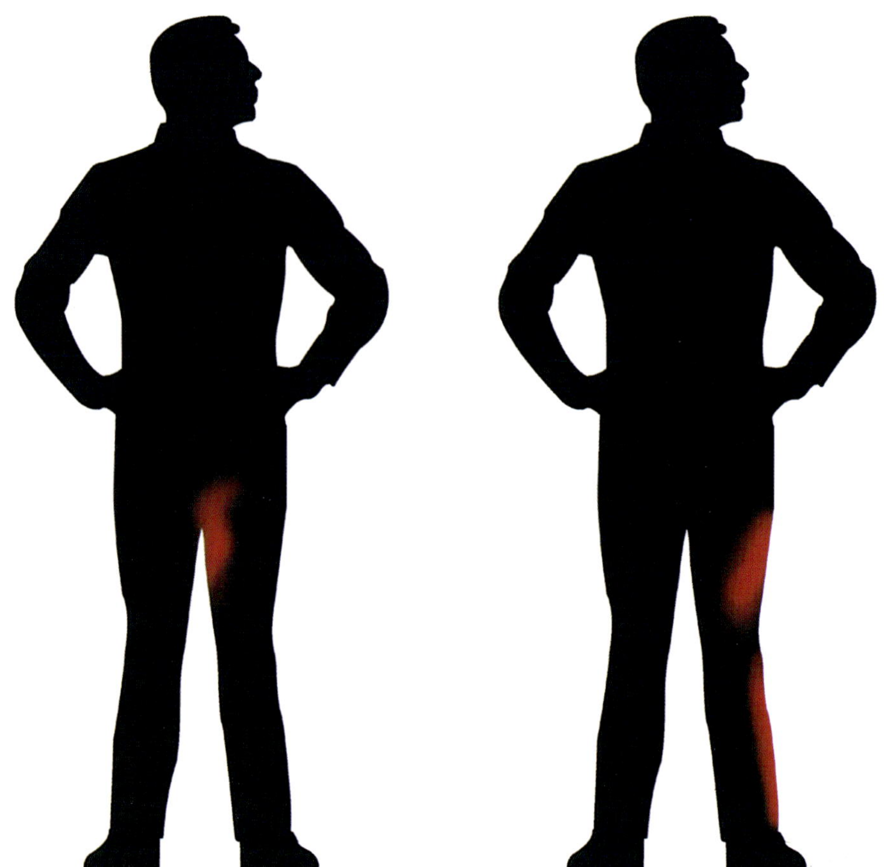

Figure 3.5
The referred pain pattern from the lower back ligaments as shown in red.

The disc

The disc is a unique structure that acts as a shock absorber and allows flexibility of the spine. If the spine was a single long bone it would crack easily with movement of the body. The disc is sandwiched between two vertebrae (bones) as shown in *Figure 3.6*.

The outside wall of the disc consists of the annular ligament (ring ligament) and the centre of the disc is made up of gel (*Figure 3.7*). The water content of the gel can be up to 90 percent. The ring ligament is composed of thin layers that are fused together. The layers are actually criss-crossed to give the ring ligament incredible strength. The top and bottom of the disc are covered by a thin plate that allows diffusion of nutrients and water into and out of the disc.

Very large forces are often transmitted onto the disc when a person performs heavy lifting, bending or twisting. The pressure inside the disc has been measured to increase ten times when someone lifts a five kilogram object. The ring ligament is thick and thought to absorb half the pressure, with the gel absorbing the other half. The disc acts like a hydraulic system. When pressure is exerted onto the gel the pressure is distributed evenly throughout the ring ligament, regardless of which way the spine bends (*Figure 3.8*).

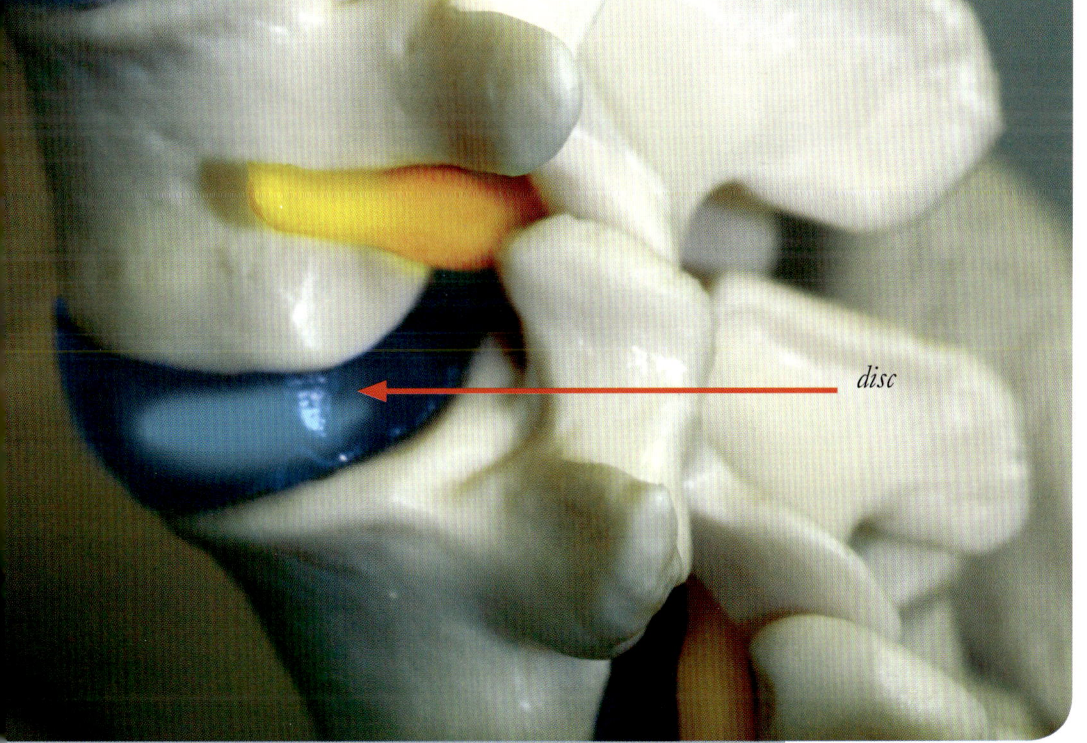

Figure 3.6
The disc is sandwiched between two vertebrae.

Figure 3.7
The disc consists of a gel centre that is surrounded by a ring ligament.

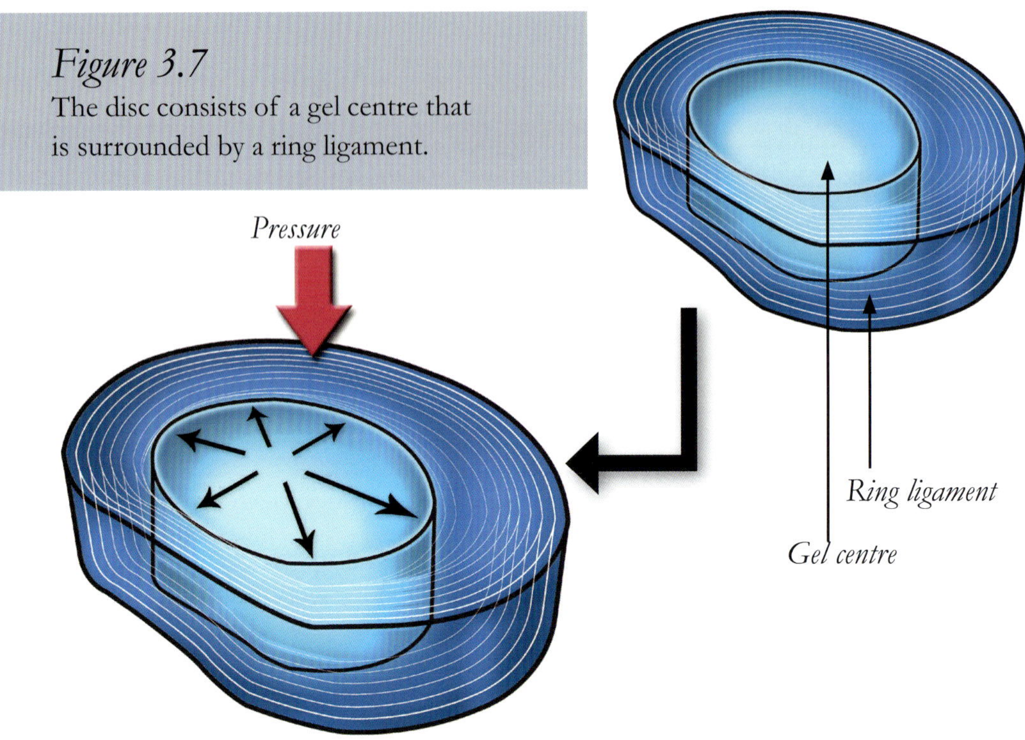

Figure 3.8
The disc acts like a hydraulic piece of machinery with the gel in the middle of the ring ligament spreading pressure to all parts of the disc wall.

On loading the disc when standing, the water within the gel can diffuse through the thin plate on the top and bottom of the disc into the adjacent bone. This causes the water in the gel to move into the adjacent bones and reduces the height of the disc as shown in *Figures 3.9* and *3.10*. When there is no loading of the disc, such as when lying down, the water returns to the gel through the thin plate (*Figure 3.11*). During the day, people may lose up to two centimetres of height due to the effect of gravity. On waking in the morning, their lost height will be restored as the water returns to the disc overnight.

Figure 3.9

The effects of pressure on the disc squeezing water out through the endplates of the adjacent vertebrae.

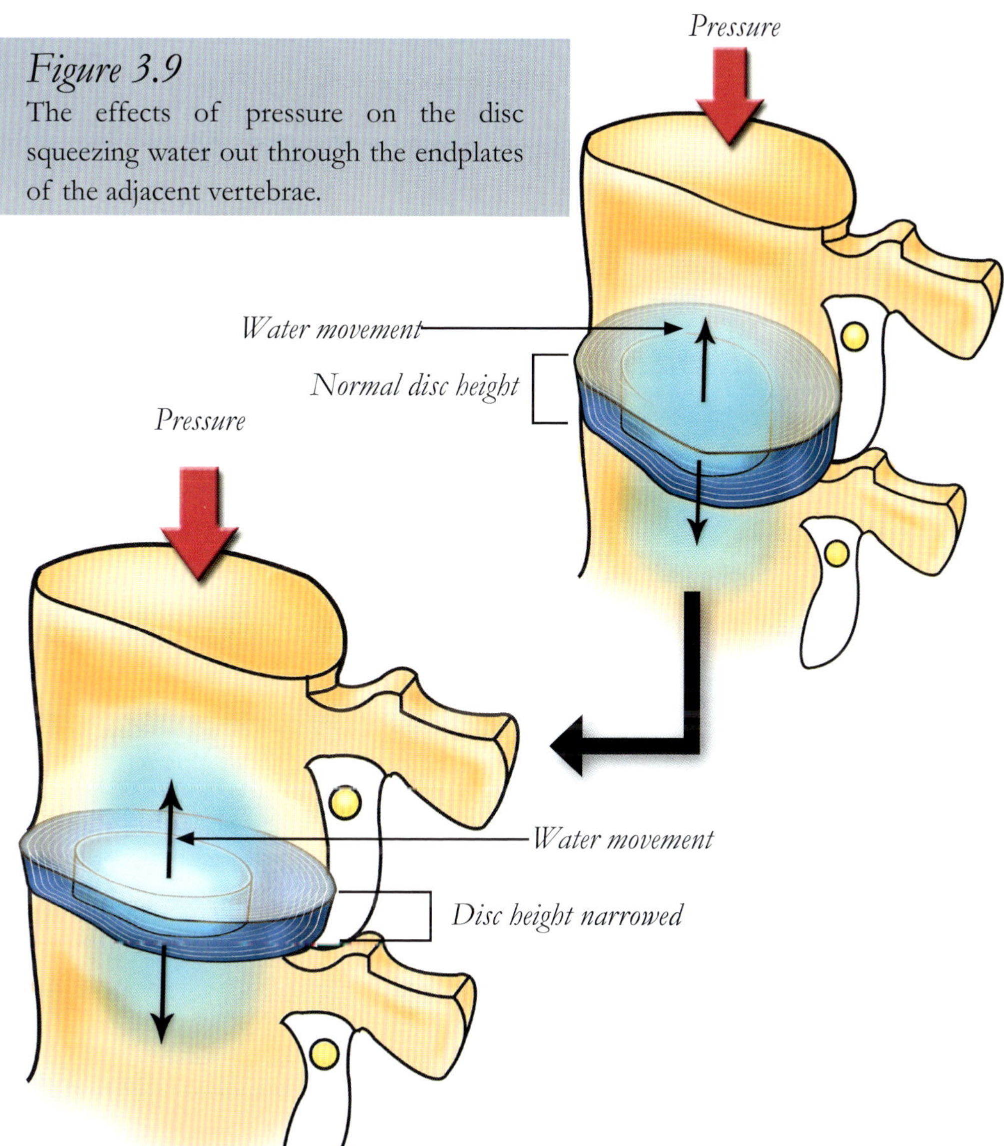

Figure 3.10

The disc narrows in the upright posture over the course of the day. Activities that load the lower back such as bending and lifting can increase the narrowing that occurs due to increased pressure on the disc.

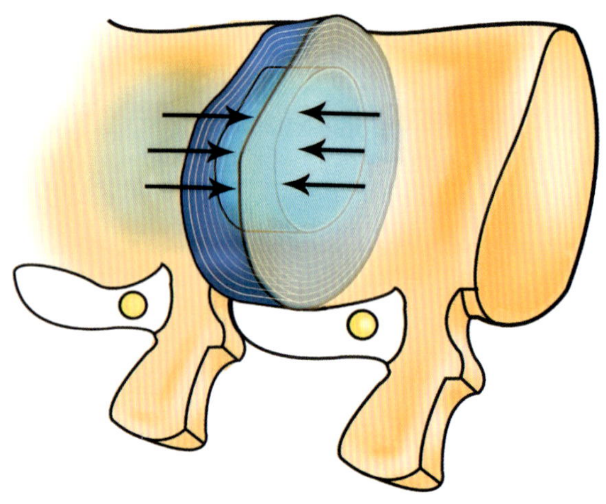

Figure 3.11
When lying down, gravity is removed and the water returns from the adjacent bones into the gel of the disc. Disc height is regained.

Although the ring ligament is very strong, it can develop tears due to accidents such as falls or motor vehicle injuries. It may even deteriorate due to poor posture. The layers of the ring ligament can separate and some of the inner layers of the ring can tear from repeated pressure. The ring ligament can therefore become filled with the gel oozing from the centre of the disc, as shown in *Figure 3.12*. The gel loses its water when entering the ring ligament, becoming dry.

So what happens to the hydraulic function of the disc once the gel becomes dry? The pressure within the gel no longer spreads evenly around the ligament. Instead the torn portion of the ring ligament is stretched, creating a disc bulge as shown in *Figure 3.13*.

A bulge can progress to the point that the entire width of the ligament develops a tear, causing the centre gel to protrude through the ring ligament, resulting in a disc prolapse (slipped disc), as shown in *Figure 3.14*.

Figure 3.12
A torn ring ligament filled with the gel.

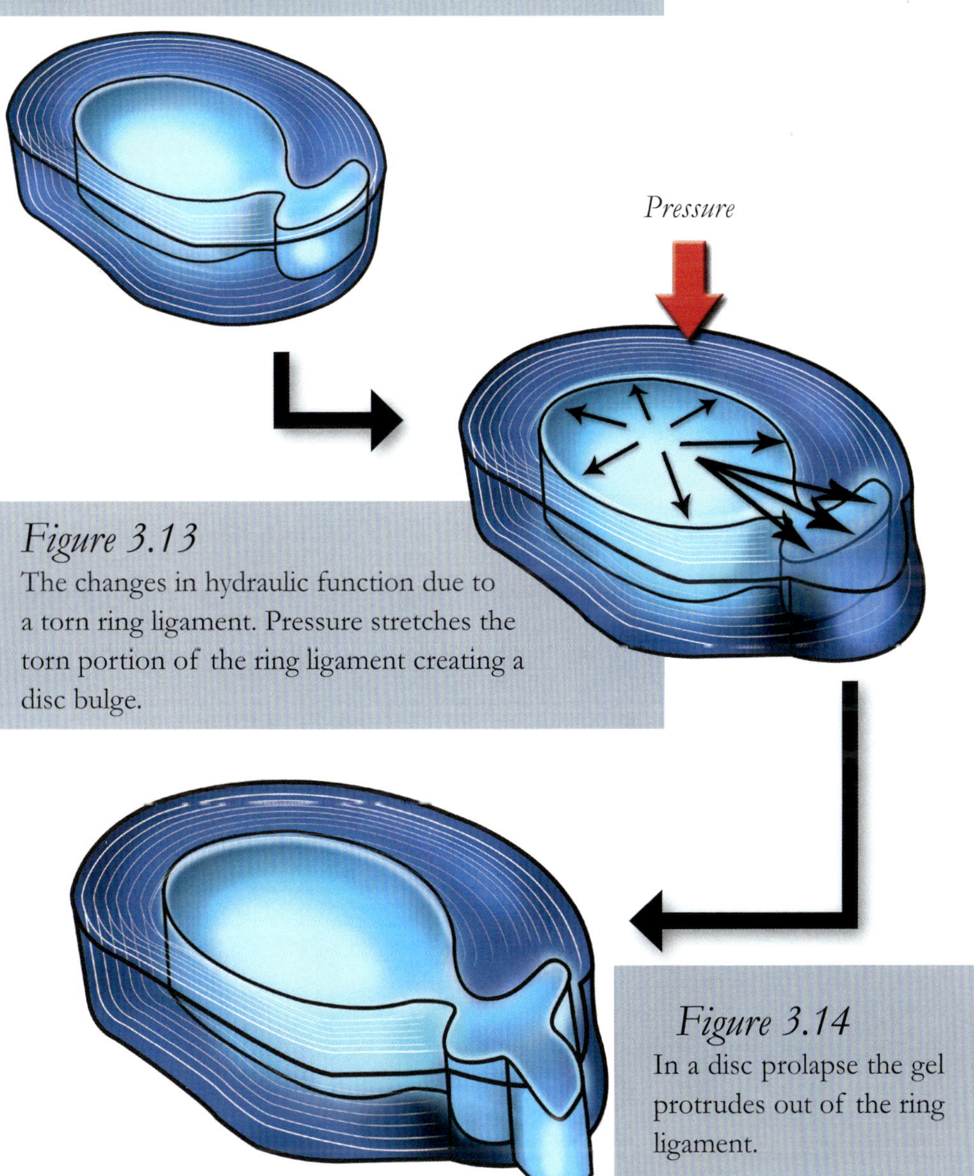

Figure 3.13
The changes in hydraulic function due to a torn ring ligament. Pressure stretches the torn portion of the ring ligament creating a disc bulge.

Figure 3.14
In a disc prolapse the gel protrudes out of the ring ligament.

A disc prolapse can cause pressure on the nerve that exits near the disc as shown in *Figure 3.15* and *3.16*. The nerves that exit the lower back are long and can extend as far as the toes. Irritation or pressure on these nerves can result in sharp, shooting severe pain as far down as the foot. These nerves control muscle power and sensation of the skin in the leg, meaning both weakness and numbness may result due to disruption of the nerve signal.

The pain suffered by those with a slipped disc pressing on a nerve is severe and has been described by women in the clinic as worse than the pain of childbirth. It would be like striking your funny bone and then keeping the funny bone pressed against a table for days, weeks or even months. If pressure continues on the nerve for long periods of time, numbness and weakness in the leg may become permanent. Fortunately, a slipped disc will usually shrink in time relieving symptoms, however patients often welcome pain relief while waiting for this improvement to occur.

Forward bending, such as vacuuming, leaning over a sink and cleaning showers, heavy lifting, twisting and sitting for long periods aggravate lower back pain as they place pressure on the discs in the lower back. Sometimes, even activities such as sneezing, coughing or bending can increase pressure in

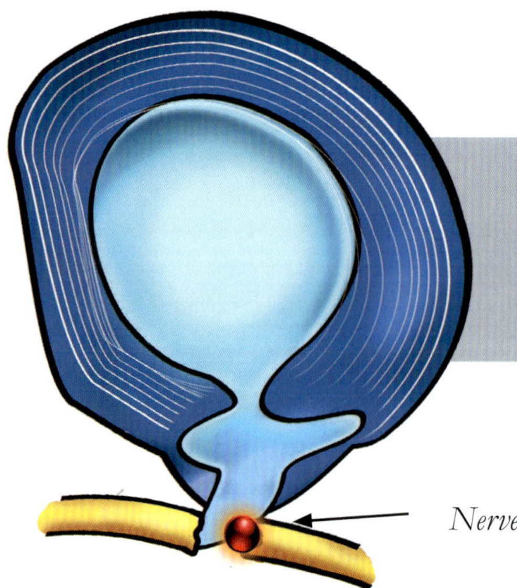

Figure 3.15
The centre gel can squeeze through the wall of the disc (disc prolapse) and irritate the nerve that travels down the leg.

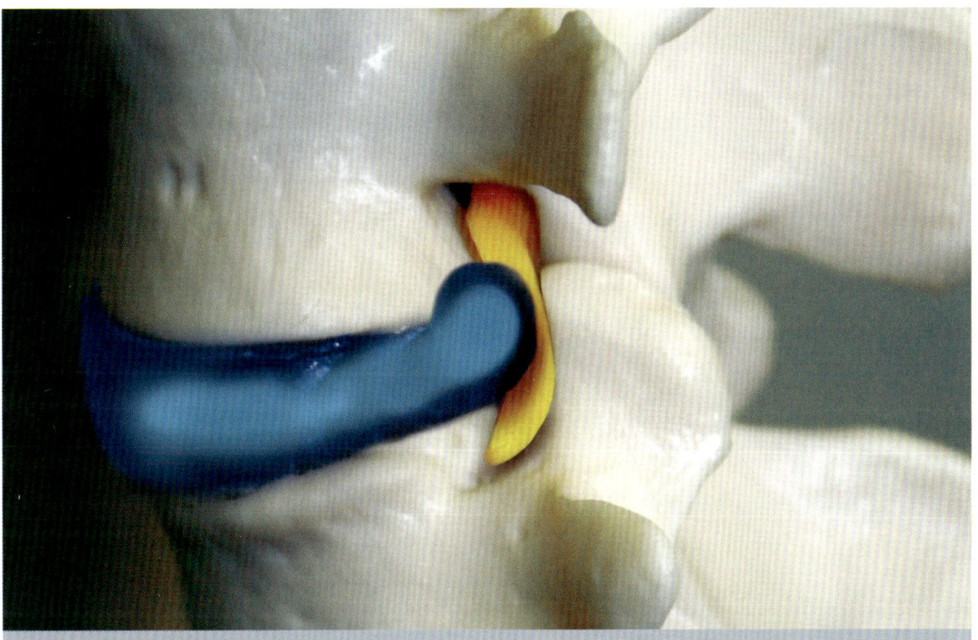

Figure 3.16
The disc prolapse is pressing and irritating the nerve that supplies the leg (yellow).

the disc and occasionally even squeeze gel out of the disc creating a slipped disc.

Often a person will injure their disc and then experience repeated episodes of back pain whenever they irritate the injured disc. In the first few years after a disc injury, disc height is maintained and X-rays show no abnormality as they only depict the bones. MRI scans, on the other hand show good disc detail and show changes in the disc structure.

Once the gel loses water, it no longer absorbs its share of the pressure, meaning the ring ligament absorbs most of the pressure and becomes squashed. After many years the disc starts to reduce in height and this can be seen on an X-ray as a narrowed gap between two vertebrae (*Figure 3.18*).

As time passes, significant changes occur in the endplate of an injured

CASE STUDY: *Andy*

Andy, a plumber by trade, was lifting a cast iron bathtub 18 years before visiting my clinic and developed sudden onset lower back pain, which radiated down his left leg. He also experienced pins and needles in the left leg that went as far as his big toe. Whenever he performed heavy lifting or prolonged bending, such as digging a trench, he would experience another episode of lower back pain. He took an anti-inflammatory whenever his lower back pain increased.

When I reviewed Andy, he knew something was wrong with his back but was unsure of the diagnosis or how to manage his pain. He had visited the physiotherapist, chiropractor, manipulative physiotherapist, Bowen therapist and seen his doctor. X-rays were taken and he was advised they were within normal limits.

Andy experienced constant lower back pain that intermittently flared up with activities. Several times a year he was bedridden for up to a few weeks because of his lower back pain.

Examination showed a loss of sensation in the left foot and marked tenderness over the lower back. Andy's previous X-rays, which he had brought along, showed disc narrowing at the lower back. I ordered a MRI scan *(Figure 3.17),* which confirmed a disc prolapse in the lower back was pressing on the nerve supplying his left leg.

An epidural injection rendered him pain-free for the next month and provided 80 percent relief for the next few months. Andy stopped taking his painkillers and began sleeping through the night. He is managing his job as a plumber, and more importantly, has learned what causes his pain, the postures that will reduce his pain, and how to perform activities such as heavy lifting and bending in a way that should not aggravate his lower back pain.

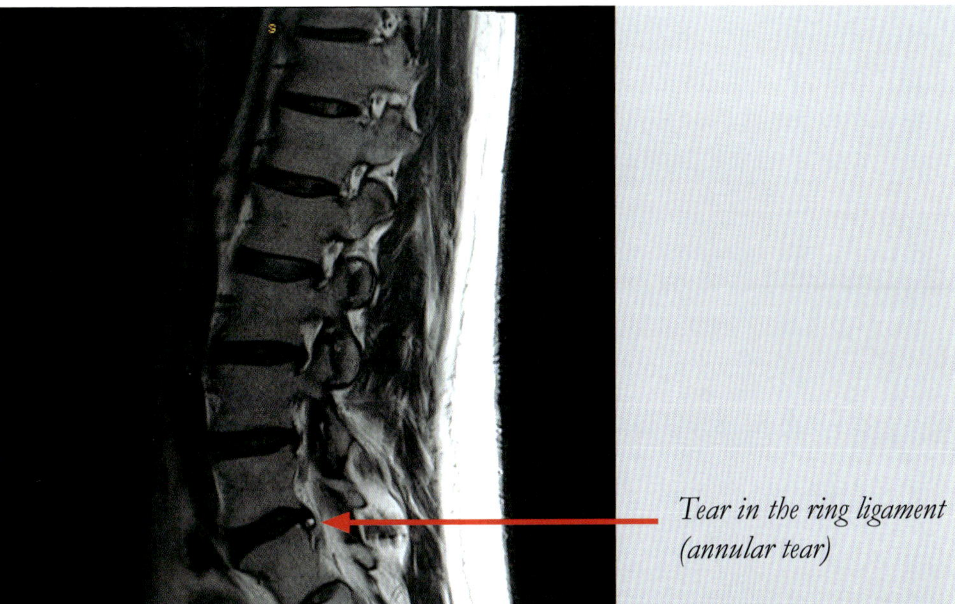

Figure 3.17
The MRI scan shows a tear in the ring ligament that appears as a white spot at the back of the disc. The white represents the fluid from the gel, which is now embedded in the ring ligament.

disc. There is a proliferation of new nerves and blood vessels in response to the extra pressure that falls on the endplate of the vertebrae. The endplate becomes more sensitive as a result of the nerves as these detect pressure, create electrical sparks which in turn is experienced as pain. Compounding the problem are the changes in the disc such as the loss of water in the gel that changes the disc from a fluid structure to a more solid structure that exerts more pressure on the vertebrae. The combination of extra nerves and a more solid disc is the most likely cause of lower back pain in the vast majority of people with lower back pain. Fortunately once a person adopts better postures that reduce pressure on the disc and tries treatments such as inversion therapy described in Chapter 5, the increased nerves are likely to subside, leaving the bones less sensitive to pressure and reducing pain.

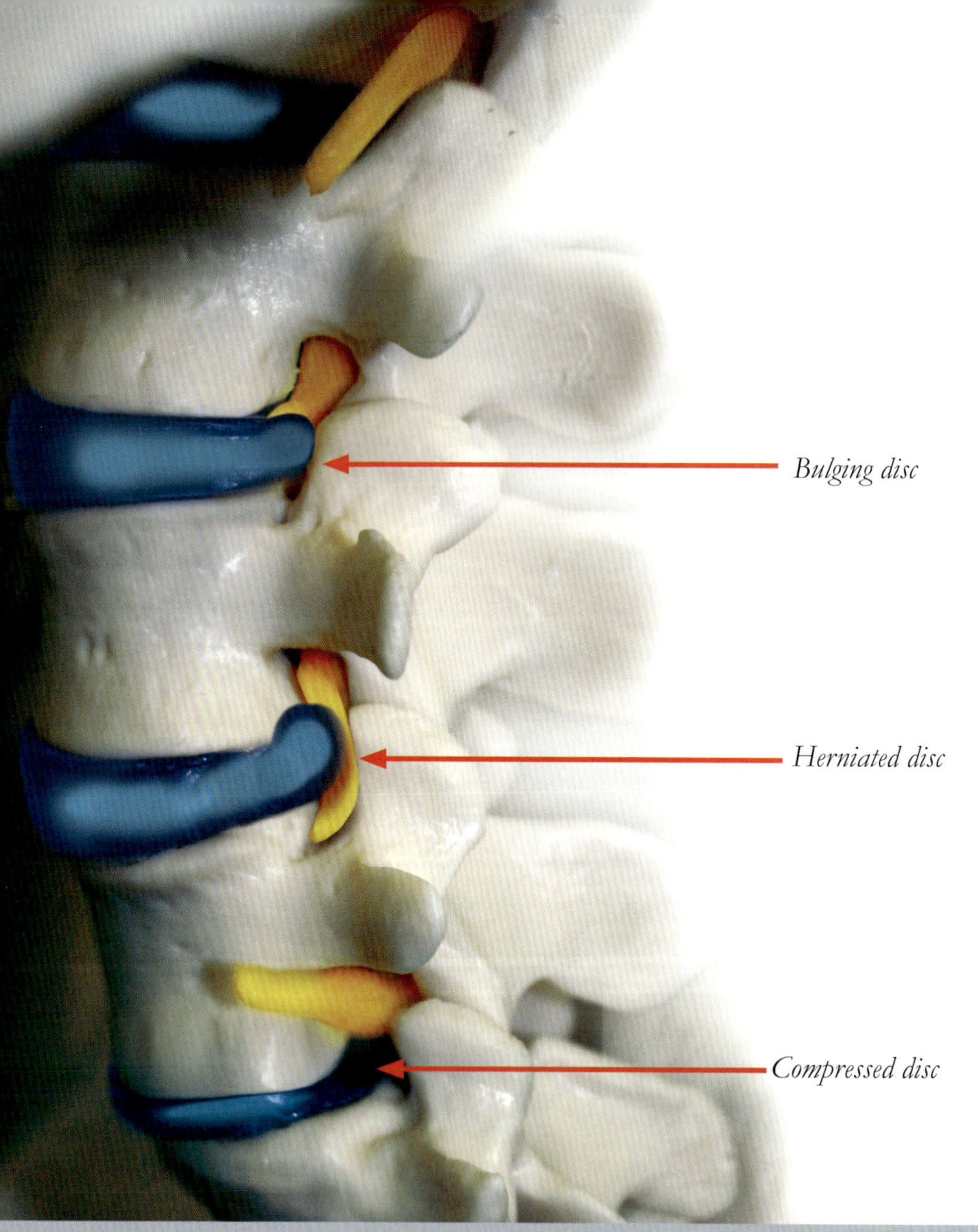

Figure 3.18

The lowest disc has lost height compared to the other levels. Once the ring ligament is torn, the gel centre no longer absorbs its share of the pressure. This means that more pressure falls on the ring ligament, squashing it over many years.

CASE STUDY: *Shane*

Shane had performed many strenuous labouring jobs since leaving school. Fifteen years before visiting my clinic he was demolishing a concrete block wall, only to find himself trapped under the concrete rubble as it collapsed. He fractured several ribs, ruptured his spleen and developed lower back pain that stopped him working.

Shane reported pain deep in his lower back and buttock region, radiating into his left leg. He experienced numbness and tingling in the left leg down to the foot. He could not even sit straight without aggravating the electrical feelings in his leg and had to sit with a lean to the right side. Walking for as little as ten minutes increased his left buttock and leg pain. Bending, lifting, crouching and sneezing also increased his symptoms.

As soon as I saw Shane it was clear that there was something damaged in his lower back. I ordered an MRI scan that showed a large prolapsed disc, as seen in *Figure 3.19.* I administered an epidural injection that alleviated his severe pain. While this improved his immediate symptoms, Shane will need to change his activities in the future, as many of them have the potential to aggravate his lower back pain and create recurrent symptoms.

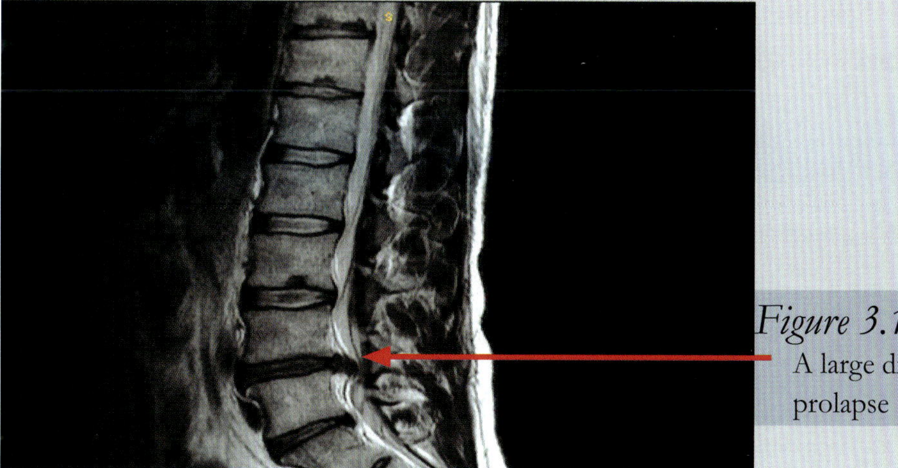

Figure 3.19
A large disc prolapse

The facet joint

The small joints that sit behind the spine are called facet joints. Occasionally these joints can be a source of lower back pain. Many studies show between five and ten percent of long-term lower back pain can be due to these joints, however the incidence of facet joint pain is thought to increase in the elderly. If the disc narrows, the joints come closer together and may press against each other, leading to pain. Pain arising from a facet joint in the lower back can also radiate down the leg, as shown in *Figure 3.21*.

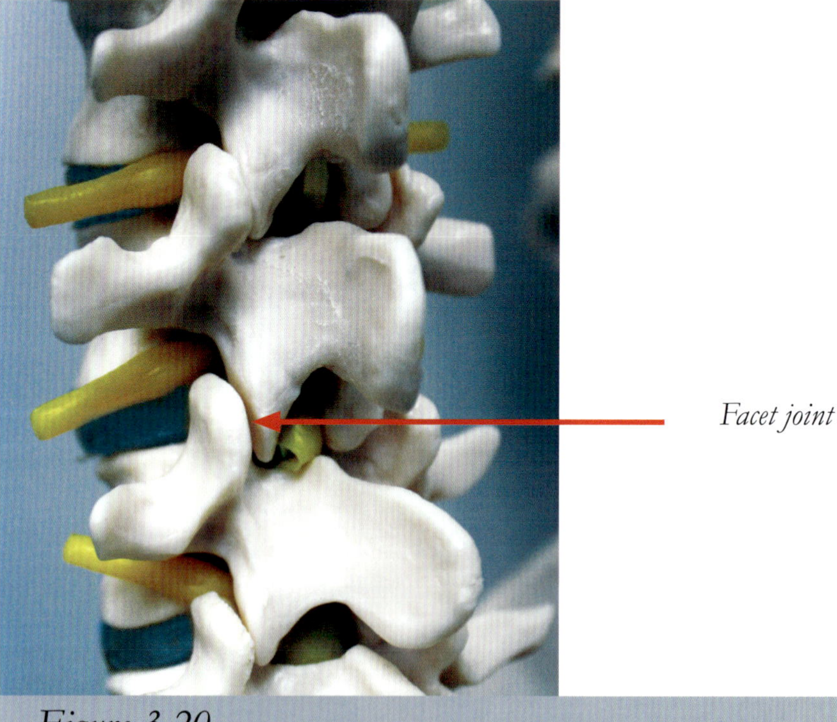

Figure 3.20
The facet joint in the lower back.

Figure 3.21

Pain arising from the facet joint can also radiate down into the leg as shown in red.

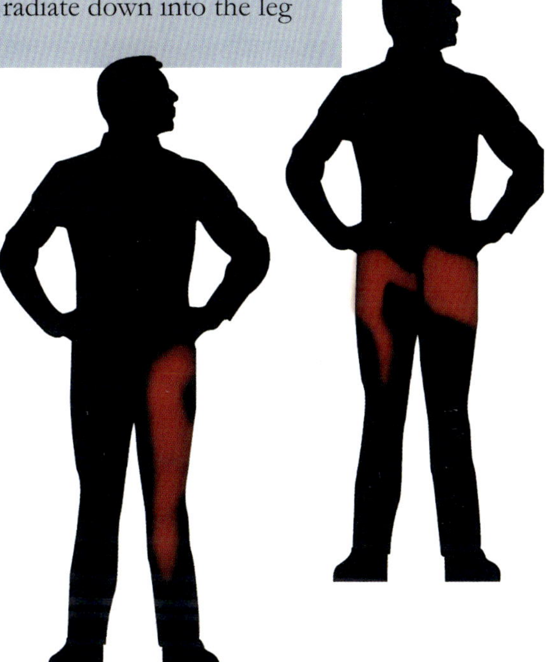

CASE STUDY: *Rangi*

Rangi, a 43-year-old woman, had suffered from constant lower back pain for four years before visiting my clinic. The pain limited running and going to the gym. Her sleep was also disturbed frequently by her pain. I injected her facet joint with a steroid under radiological guidance. When I reviewed her several weeks later, all of her symptoms had resolved and she had returned to running and attending the gym.

Although the injection provided good relief, it was likely that Rangi's pain would return as the steroid wore off. I phoned her two years later and she was still happy with the results of the injection. She was also very pleased to know the likely source of her symptoms.

CASE STUDY: *Matthew*

Matthew developed lower back and left leg pain after he skidded and landed on his side during a motorcycle accident. The pain in his left leg was sharp and shooting and was accompanied by pins and needles.

Matthew worked as a chef, and lifting heavy pots and bending over the sink aggravated his symptoms. An MRI scan confirmed my suspicion that a disc prolapse was causing his pain, as shown in *Figure 3.22*. A large disc prolapse was compressing the nerve that supplied Matthew's left leg, hence the shooting pain in his leg.

Matthew's scan revealed an interesting feature: a narrow disc at the lowest part of the lower back. In this case, the variation in his spine was not the cause of his symptoms.

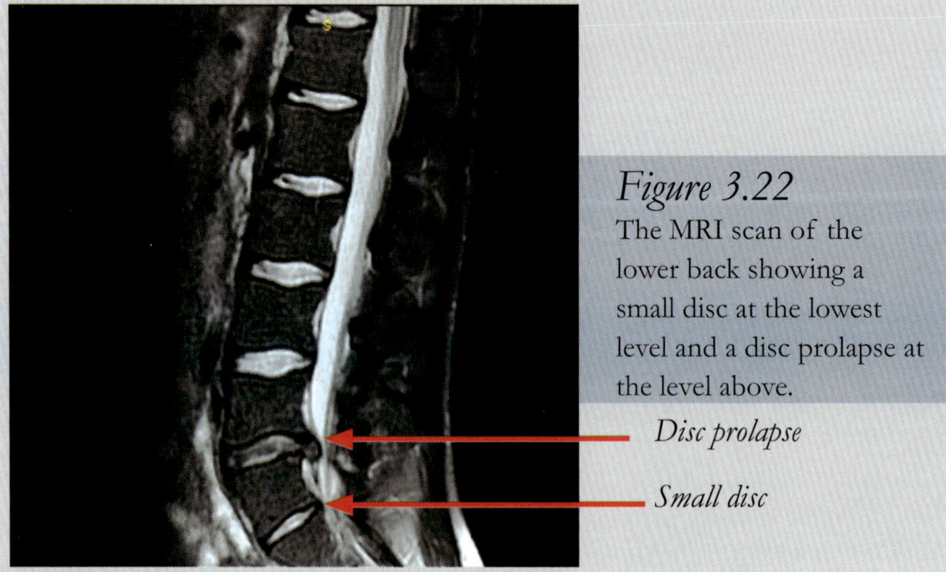

Figure 3.22
The MRI scan of the lower back showing a small disc at the lowest level and a disc prolapse at the level above.

Variations of the spine

Sometimes, performing an X-ray will reveal differences from the normal arrangement of the lower back such as six lower back vertebrae instead of the usual five, an extension of the vertebrae can touch the pelvic bones, or even the lowest vertebra is fused to the sacrum. Such abnormalities can occasionally be the source of pain.

The hip

Problems in the hip can cause buttock and leg pain, as shown in *Figure 3.23*. Between October 2008 and June 2009, over 40 patients presented to my clinic with lower back pain and significant hip problems. The hip joint is a ball and socket joint, and the hip bone is the outermost part of the thigh. Any fall onto the side or even back can cause the ball to hit the socket. This can result in injury to the hip joint. Hip pain is usually felt in the groin region.

In patients who experience lower back pain, the hip is usually excluded as a source of pain by taking a detailed history of their complaints, examining the hips and ordering appropriate investigations. If pain is made worse by walking, getting off a chair after sitting for long periods, getting into and out of a car, walking up or down stairs or inclines and running, it may point to the hip joint.

There is sometimes significant confusion diagnosing hip pain from lower back and sacro-iliac joint pain, as the same activities can aggravate pain and the spread of pain into the buttock and leg can be similar. In one patient, a hernia operation was performed, and in another patient, a testicular release operation was performed when both patients suffered from hip pain.

Investigations such as X-rays of the hip are usually within normal limits unless advanced changes are present. MRI scans show better detail of the ball and socket when a diagnosis is in doubt.

Treatment of hip pain can include refraining from activities that aggravate pain, such as prolonged walking or running. Strengthening the gluteal muscles (as shown in *Figure 3.24)* can help maintain a better alignment of the hips. Stretches for the hip flexor muscles (as shown in *Figure 3.25)* can also be useful. A steroid injection into the hip joint may alleviate pain.

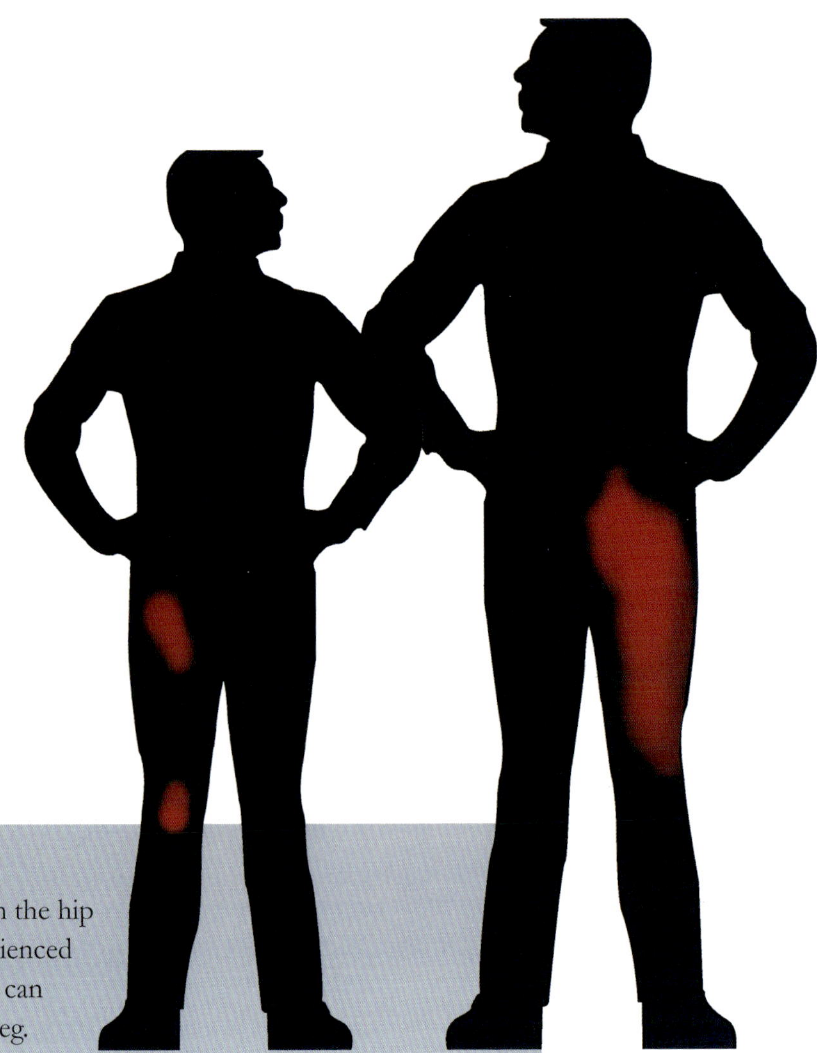

Figure 3.23
Pain arising from the hip is typically experienced in the groin, but can radiate into the leg.

Figure 3.24
Strengthening of the gluteal muscles.

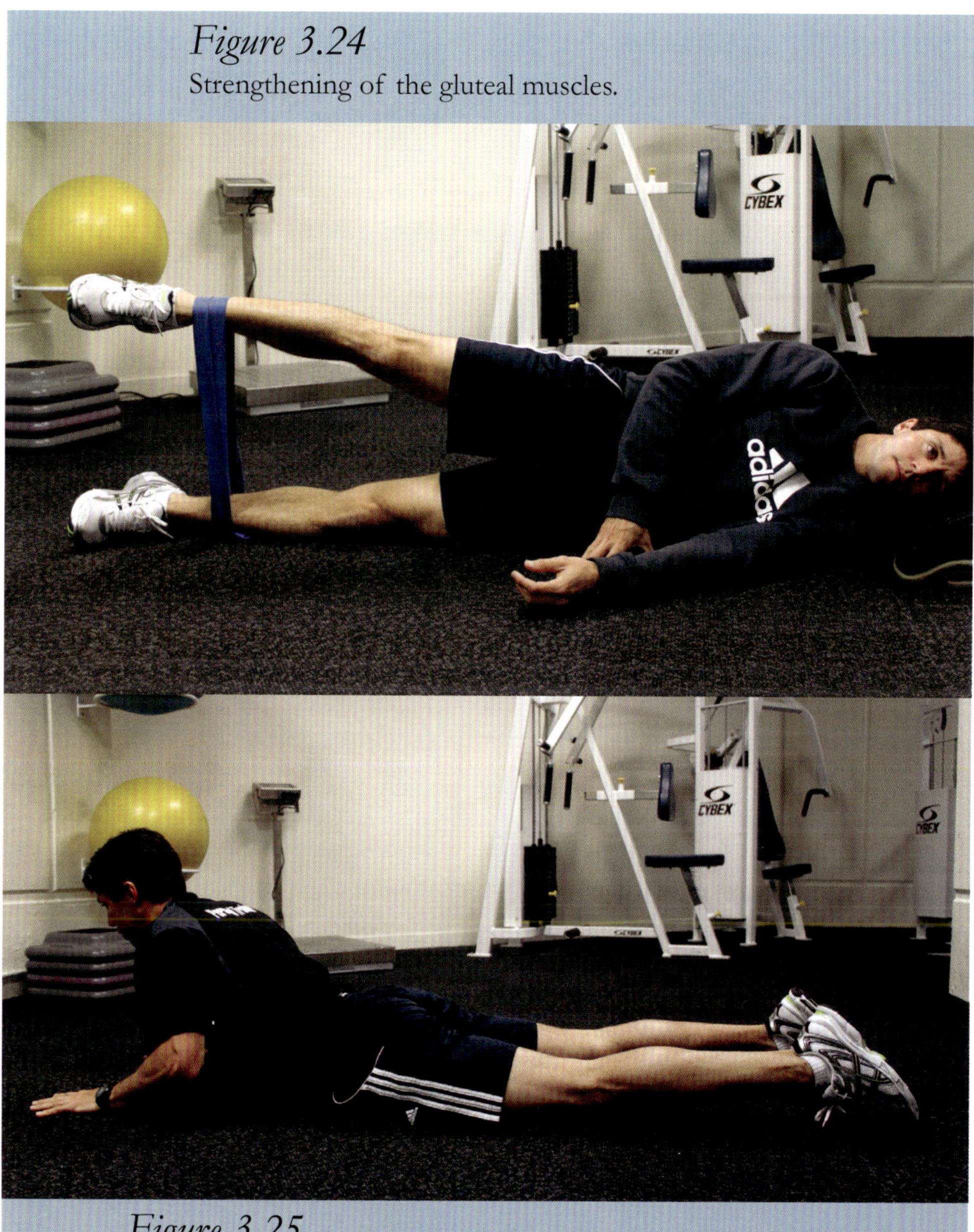

Figure 3.25
A stretch for the hip flexor muscles.

CASE STUDY: *Brian*

Brian, aged 35, fell of his mountain bike, landing on his left side. He experienced only mild immediate pain but recalled waking the next day, unable to get out of bed due to lower back pain. Over the following six years his symptoms had increased and affected his ability to play with his young children, play sport and sit at his desk for long periods. The pain was a constant ache and annoyed him greatly.

Brian went to physiotherapy with some improvement, but a year after his initial injury went for a run that made his back pain worse. He was referred to a spinal surgeon. X-rays and a MRI scan *(Figure 3.26)* of the lower back were within normal limits. He attended a back institute but even after nine months of intensive therapy his pain continued to trouble him. He had taken several medications including Vioxx, Panadeine, diclofenac, Codral Forte, Tramadol and diazepam. He had also visited a chiropractor but in the last session developed a migraine.

I reviewed Brian five years after his initial injury, and examination revealed good movement of the lower back with marked tenderness over the hip muscles. Moving the left hip in certain directions caused pain. The muscles surrounding the hip and back were treated and Brian's pain localised to the left hip. I ordered an MRI scan of his left hip *(Figure 3.27)* that showed the hip was the likely cause of his pain.

Brian underwent keyhole surgery of the hip which improved his pain to the point where he was able to kick a soccer ball with his kids. He reduced his painkillers three months after the operation. He was surprised that the hip was the source of his symptoms as he had always thought it was his lower back. After a few years he required a hip replacement as his pain returned. The hip replacement was successful in alleviating most of his symptoms.

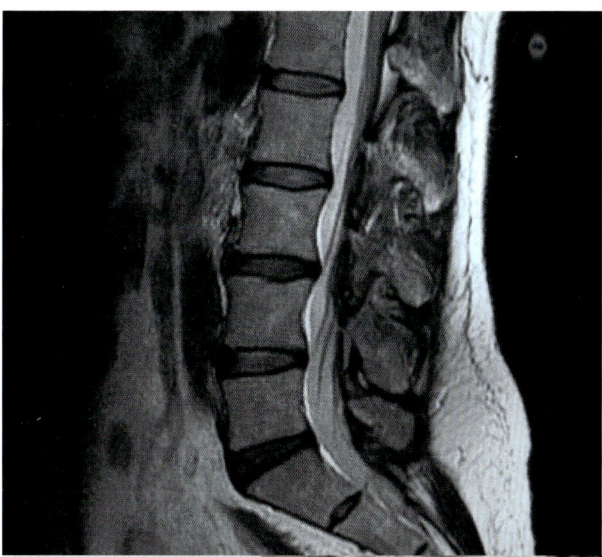

Figure 3.26
The MRI scan shows good disc heights and no significant changes in the discs of the lower back.

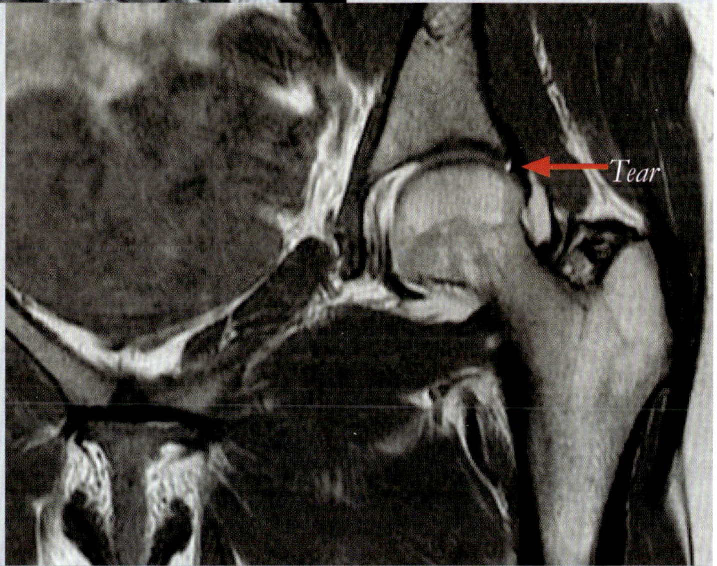

Figure 3.27
The MRI scan showing a tear of the lip of the hip socket and changes to the lining of the bones.

CASE STUDY: *Lucia*

Lucia had a motorcycle accident when she slid on gravel and landed on her left side. She sustained a fracture of her upper back and also experienced lower back and left leg pain. Lucia was unable to continue her work as a nurse and found an office position that did not involve heavy lifting.

Although heavy lifting, repeated bending and sitting for long periods aggravated her symptoms, walking was Lucia's greatest limitation and she needed crutches to leave the house. Her sleep was disturbed and she was feeling depressed as a result of the pain and the limitations it was putting on her life. She had started taking several medications including Prozac, Imovane, clonazepam and Nurofen with little relief.

I can recall Lucia walking into the consulting room with an obvious limp. Moving the hip exacerbated her symptoms. I advised her that her left hip was the likely source of her pain and sent her for an MRI scan that confirmed my suspicion. When anaesthetic was injected into her hip, the pain disappeared for a short time. Lucia was treated with keyhole surgery to the left hip with excellent results and returned to most activities.

The sacro-iliac joint

The sacro-iliac joint (commonly called the SI joint), as shown in *Figure 3.28,* is a very complex joint located at the base of the spinal column. There is one sacro-iliac joint on each side of the spine. Pain from the sacro-iliac joint is often experienced around the joint and into the leg, as seen in *Figure 3.29.* The sacro-iliac joint is best thought of as a tectonic plate that makes small movements that protect the pelvis from cracking. The joint is held together with large ligaments and is very strong.

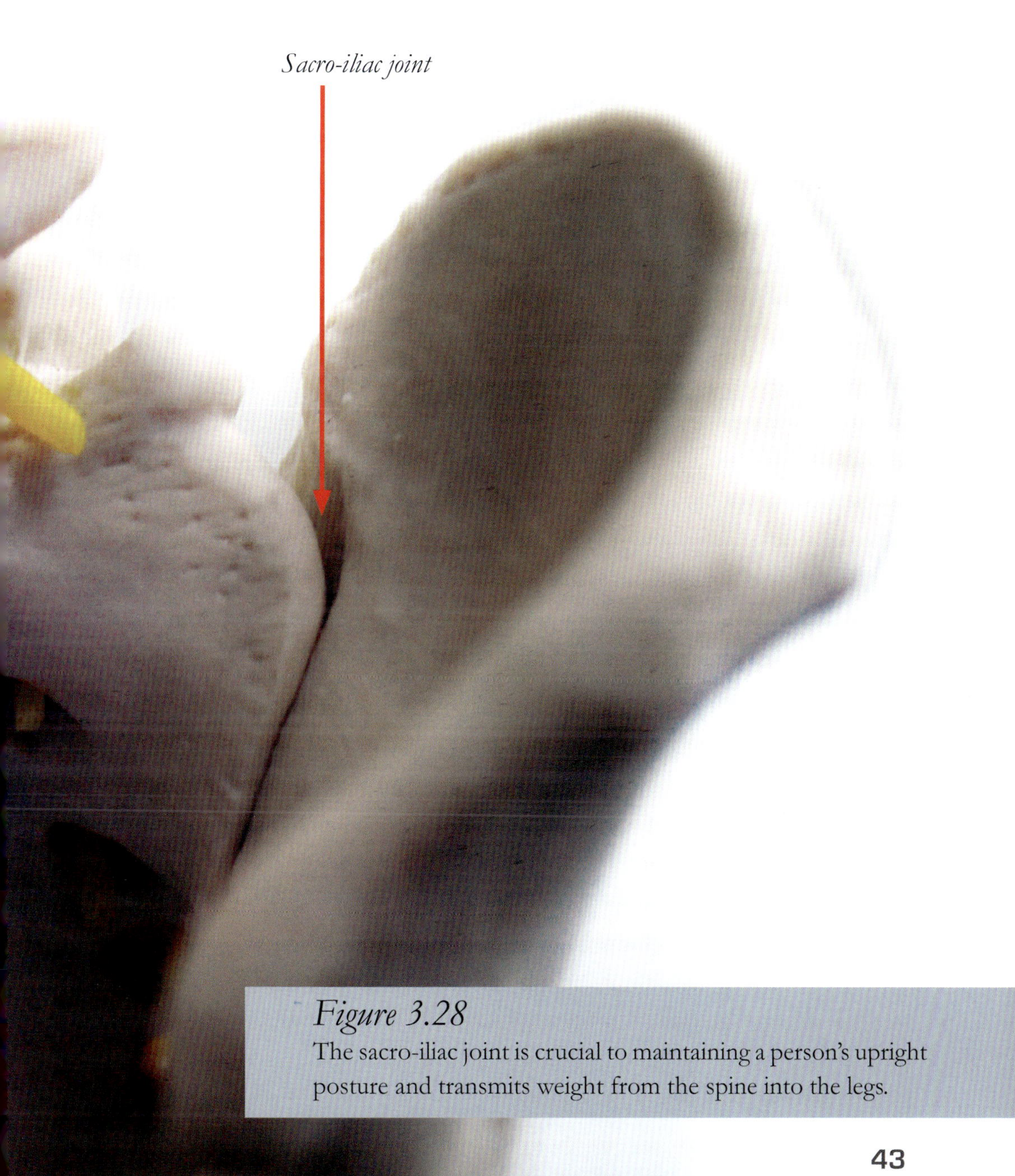

Figure 3.28
The sacro-iliac joint is crucial to maintaining a person's upright posture and transmits weight from the spine into the legs.

Pain in the buttock region is often diagnosed as SI joint pain. However, I have found there is considerable confusion between the hip, lower back and the SI joint, as all these structures can cause similar patterns of pain into the leg.

To diagnose the SI joint as a source of pain, an injection of anaesthetic can be placed under X-ray control into the joint. If the pain subsides with anaesthetic, then the joint may be the source of pain. Unfortunately, there is little treatment that consistently alleviates SI joint pain in the long term. Mobilisation, manipulation and steroid injection may offer some relief.

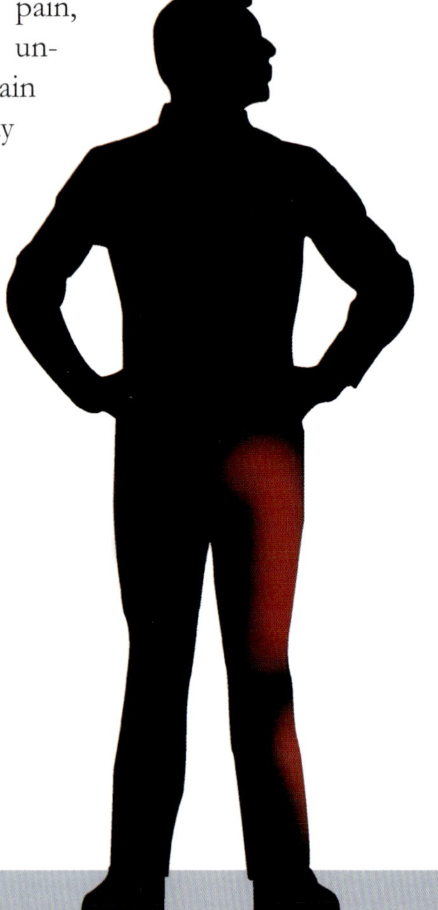

Figure 3.29

The pattern of pain from the sacro-iliac joint is usually described as being in the buttock region and can radiate down the leg.

CASE STUDY: *Emma-Jane*

In 1987, the car *Emma-Jane* was driving was hit from behind by another vehicle. The heavy impact damaged her car beyond repair. The accident left her suffering from neck, lower back and buttock pain. She also developed an irritated bladder, causing her to pass water up to five times per night. Standing or sitting increased her pain and she limped when walking for long distances.

Emma-Jane's pain had spread throughout her body and at one stage she even believed she had suffered a stroke. She had headaches, her sleep was always disturbed and she was constantly tired.

Over the years, Emma-Jane had tried several treatments. She attended the pain management team at the local hospital and even went to a specialist pain management centre twice for three-week live-in programmes. She was told that the pain was due to parts of her brain misfiring. She also attended a back institute.

Investigations, including scans of the right shoulder, liver, pelvis, sinuses and head, as well as X-rays and an MRI of the entire spine, did not show a cause for Emma-Jane's pain. She had not returned to full time work since her accident. Her depression and pain were so overwhelming that she had tried to end her life twice.

Emma-Jane tried a new infrared heat therapy in 2012 and found her pain had localised to her lower back and buttock region. After going through the history and scans, the right sacro-iliac joint was injected under CT scan. She had a marked improvement of her back pain for the first time since her accident and reduced her painkillers considerably. The sacro-iliac joint was pinpointed as the likely source of Emma-Jane's pain.

Finally understanding the cause of her symptoms alleviated a lot of Emma-Jane's distress and reassured her that it was not all in her head.

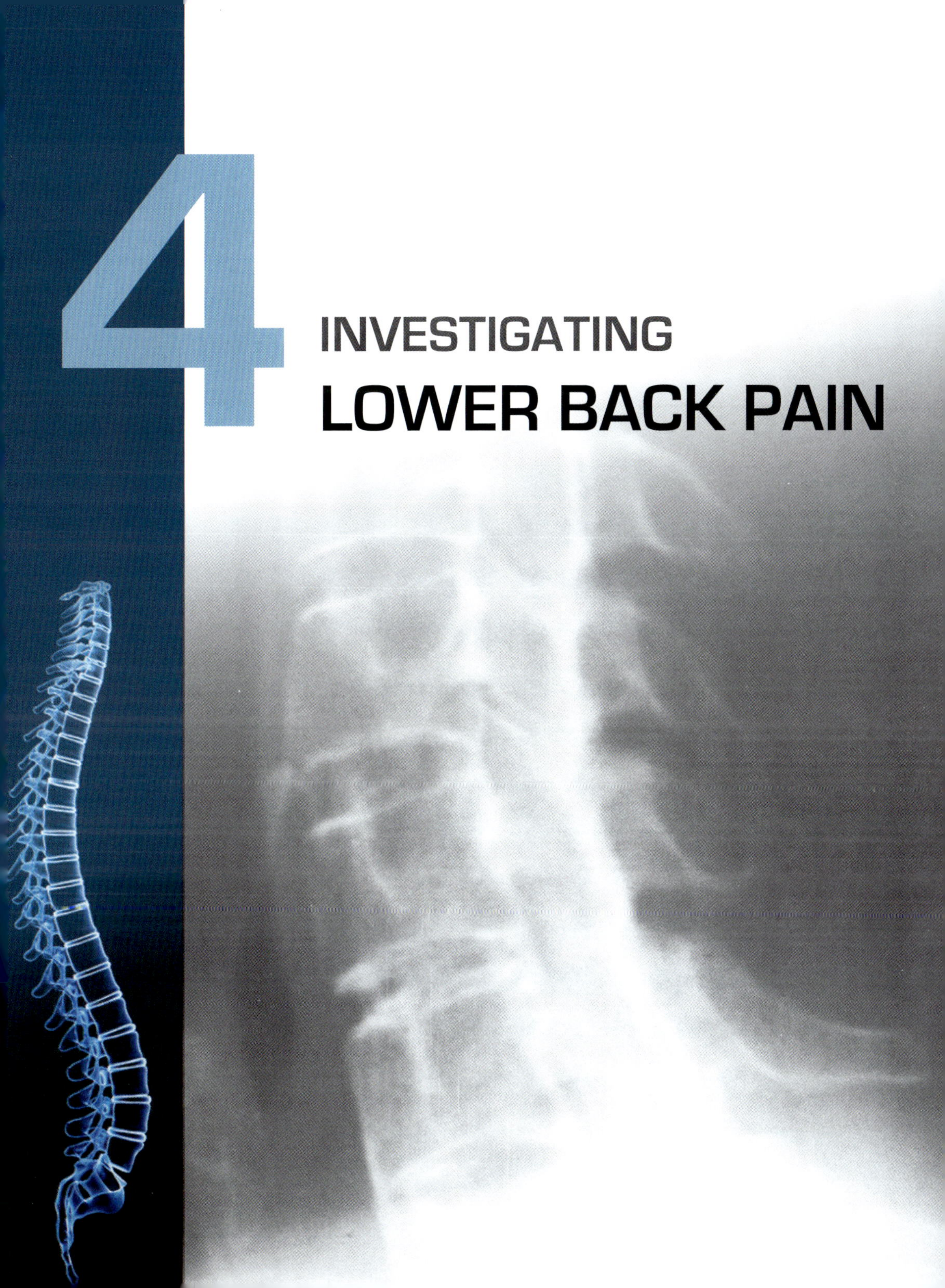

4 INVESTIGATING LOWER BACK PAIN

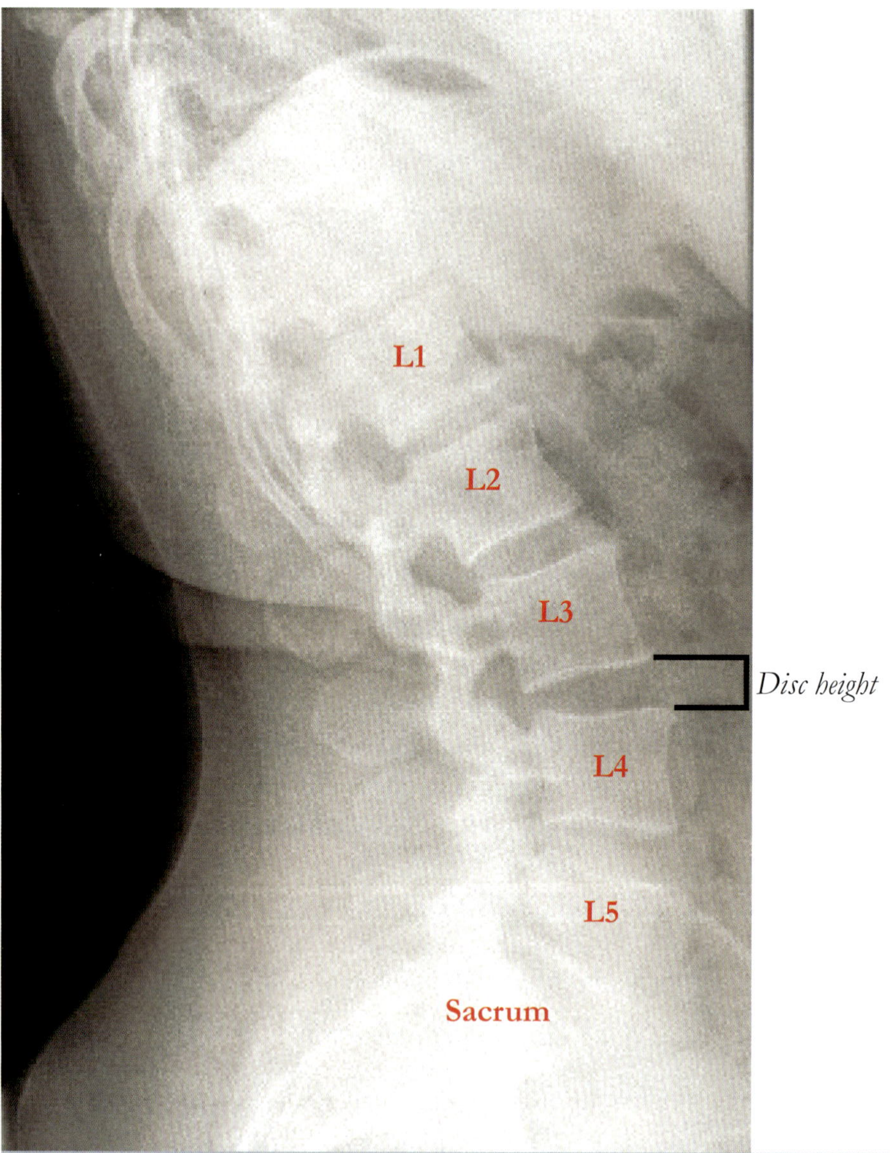

Figure 4.1

X-rays of the lower back show the bones and leave a gap where the disc is located.

Investigations are performed to see which structure is damaged and might be causing pain. Although investigations are useful, they must be interpretated with caution as they can pick up abnormalities that are not related to the pain. The most common investigations performed for lower back pain include X-ray, CT scan, MRI scan and bone scan.

X-ray

X-rays of the lower back show the bones. They are useful when looking for fractures, especially for patients who have had trauma such as a fall. X-rays may show variations present since birth and facet joint changes. An X-ray of the lower back gives an appreciation of disc height but does not show the structural details of the disc. The disc merely appears as a gap between two vertebrae. *Figure 4.1* shows a lower back X-ray. A normal X-ray does not mean you have no damage to your spine, as the disc is the most commonly damaged structure and is not well shown by an X-ray.

X-rays give off radiation. The amount of radiation exposure for a lower back X-ray is approximately 50 times the radiation from a chest X-ray, so this investigation should normally be performed when looking for fractures that are a result of trauma.

CASE STUDY: *Kona*

Kona developed lower back pain when he lifted a heavy box above his head five years before visiting my clinic. Playing lawn bowls aggravated his pain as did twisting, lifting and sitting for long periods. Fortunately, Kona worked in an office and was not limited in his work, however his part-time massage therapy work irritated his symptoms.

Examination revealed some tenderness over Kona's lower back muscles. He also had loss of sensation in the left leg, which is a sign of nerve compression. A new X-ray of the lower back was ordered and compared to an X-ray from the time of the injury, both are shown in *Figure 4.2*. It was apparent that the lowest lower back disc was approximately 20 percent narrower in the later X-ray.

I advised Kona that this disc was the likely source of his pain and provided education about the function of the disc and how to avoid placing significant pressure on it. I also recommended that Kona start swimming four to five times a week for exercise. He'd had two knee replacements and his activity levels had dropped, contributing to weight gain.

Kona returned in a month's time. He had started swimming regularly and changed his postures, with a considerable improvement in his lower back pain. He did not require an MRI scan or any further imaging, as the X-rays gave a clue to the source of his pain.

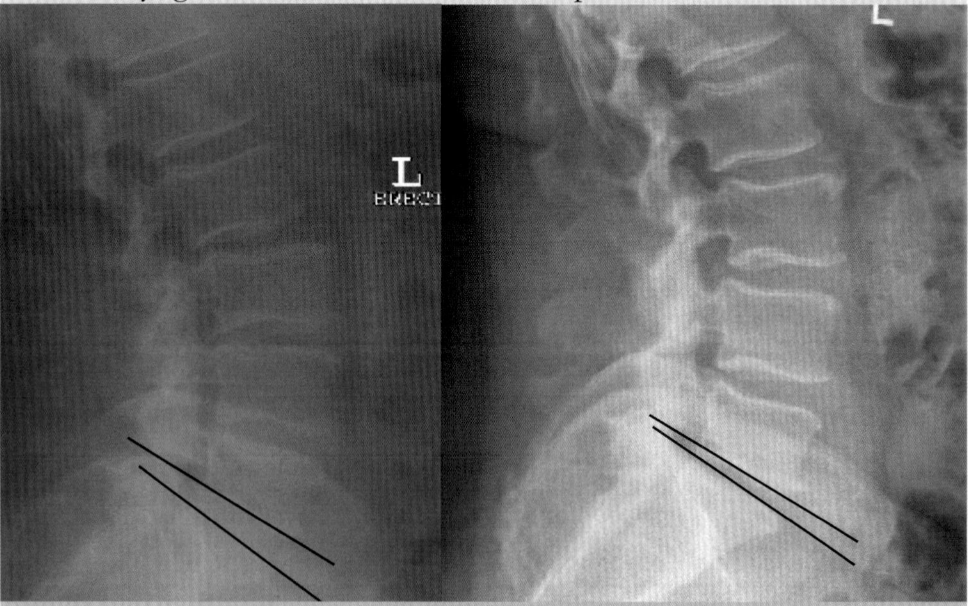

Figure 4.2

The right-hand X-ray taken five years after the left-hand X-ray shows the lowest disc space in the lower back has narrowed in the time elapsed.

Magnetic resonance imaging (MRI)

A magnetic resonance imaging (MRI) scan produces high-quality images of soft tissues such as the disc.

MRI scans use magnetic fields and do not subject the patient to radiation. A magnet is placed close to the bodysite being scanned. The scanner only takes a picture of the part of the body requested (e.g. shoulder, neck or lower back). An MRI scan does not routinely take an image of the whole body.

A disadvantage of MRI is that the scanner can be claustrophobic and emits a hammering sound.

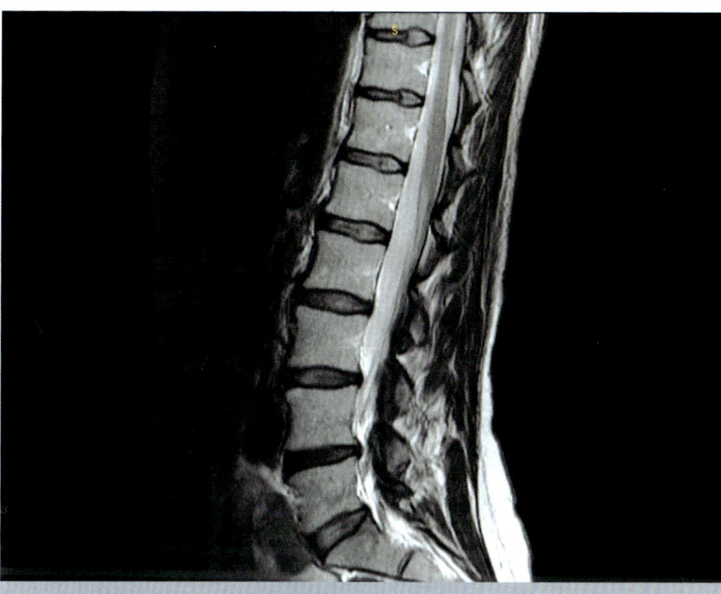

Figure 4.3
The MRI scan gives detailed information about the soft tissues, including the disc.

CASE STUDY: *Craig*

When carrying a heavy aluminium window down some steps, *Craig* twisted his lower back, resulting in pain that increased over several months as he continued working. He was becoming disabled in most activities, including prolonged sitting, walking, standing and repeated heavy lifting. He had also given up mountain running, but was keen to stay fit and managed to get to the gym most days.

An X-ray was taken, as shown in *Figure 4.4,* which showed the disc heights had reduced in the lower back. The problems were confirmed by a MRI scan *(Figure 4.5),* which also showed details of disc protrusions.

I advised Craig that repeated pressure on these discs can cause pain, and over many years can lead to disc narrowing. Craig took heed of the advice and stopped working in his manual job, shifting towards management. He also altered his posture, ensuring that he kept the curve in his back when he sat. He continued going to the gym and performing activities that did not aggravate his pain. Craig needed pain relief for several months while his pain settled.

Six months later, he was back to mountain running and had just completed a 35 kilometre mountain run when I last reviewed him. He was sleeping well and managing most activities but remained wary of repeated heavy lifting and bending. Craig shows that, despite significant changes in the discs, once you know what's going on you can often modify activity and reduce symptoms significantly.

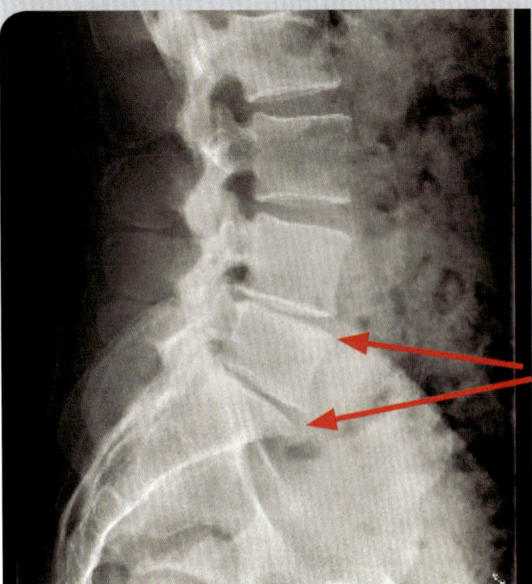

Figure 4.4
This lower back X-ray shows narrowing at the bottom two disc spaces.

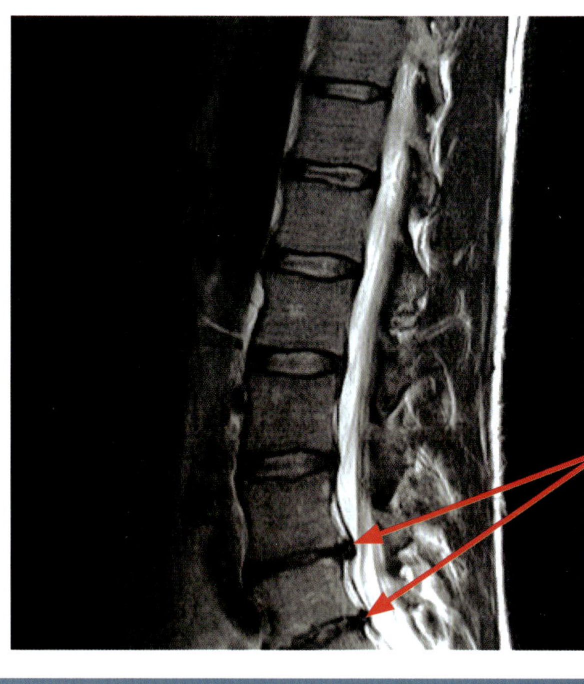

Figure 4.5
An MRI scan showing the loss of height at the bottom two discs as well as reduced gel in the centre of the discs.

Computed tomography (CT)

A computed tomography (CT) scan is like a super X-ray and gives much finer detail about bones than a standard X-ray, as seen in *Figure 4.6*. It is the most useful imaging technique for the health professional looking for precise information about a patient's bone. A trade off for this precision is increased radiation; the radiation dose of one CT scan is equivalent to 5,000 chest X-rays.

Bone scan

A bone scan *(Figure 4.7)* is a nuclear scan that detects bone that is trying to heal. It is useful to diagnose bony cancers and detect stress fractures that do not show up on normal X-rays. The patient receives an injection containing a radioactive solution that is then detected by a camera. The patient is exposed to small amounts of radiation during this test.

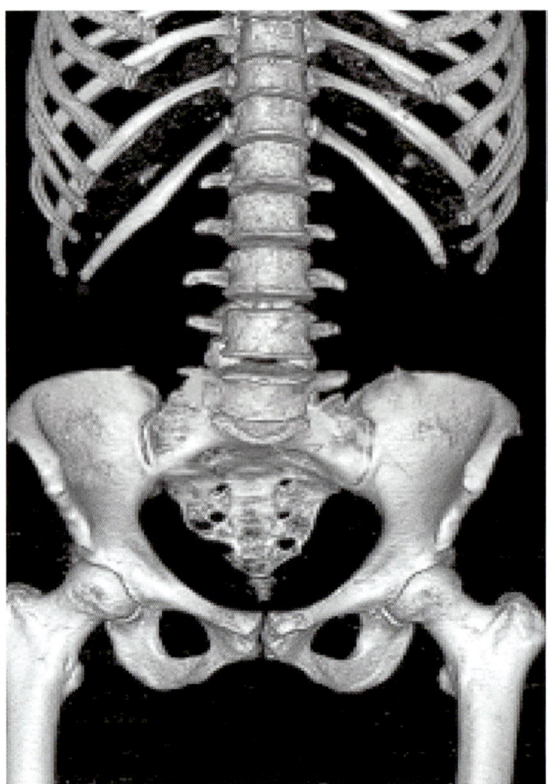

Figure 4.6
The CT scan shows bones in excellent detail.

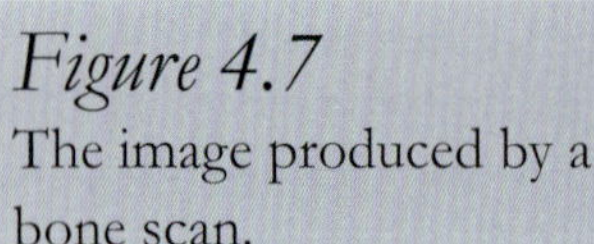

Figure 4.7
The image produced by a bone scan.

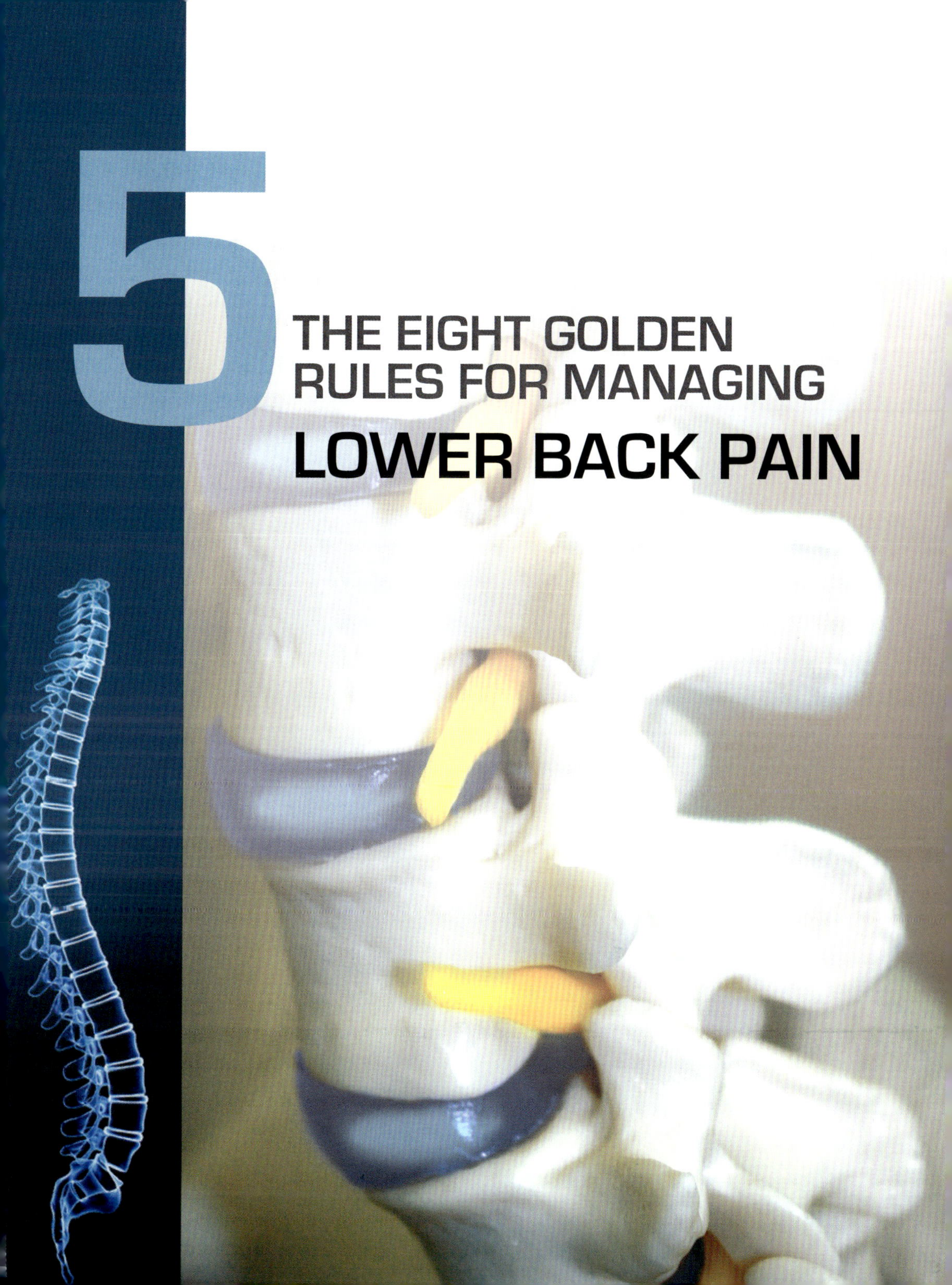

5 THE EIGHT GOLDEN RULES FOR MANAGING LOWER BACK PAIN

Managing lower back pain

This chapter outlines the eight golden rules for lower back pain. The advice is designed to alleviate pressure on the lower back discs which are the most common source of lower back pain. If activities and postures that aggravate pain are continued, then unnecessary pressure is being applied to the lower back discs. This will result in gradual narrowing of the discs and lead to a point of no return, when simple measures will no longer help your symptoms. Hence it is important to listen to your body and use the knowledge to maintain good back health. The advice is simple and self-directed.

If you have just developed lower back pain, the best thing is not to worry as most episodes of lower back pain subside within a week. It is advisable to continue normal activities as best you can, but avoid activities that aggravate pain. When pain continues, it is important to ensure that you do not damage the injured structure further by modifying activities and postures as well as perform activities that help the pain.

1. Avoid heavy lifting

You should not lift very heavy or awkward items once you have developed lower back pain. Like any injury, your back may need time to heal and is less likely to heal if reinjured, especially in the first few months after injury. If you have to lift, it is sensible to do so in piecemeal fashion. Carrying multiple light loads rather than a few heavier loads will help to protect your back from further injury and reduce recurrences of lower back pain. Bending and twisting repeatedly can also perpetuate a disc injury and prevent healing.

2. Maintain the lower back curve

The word lordosis refers to the curved shape of the lower back, as shown in *Figure 5.1*. The lower back is not a straight column because the building blocks (vertebrae and discs) are not square. Instead, the vertebrae and discs

CASE STUDY: *Barry*

When *Barry,* an accountant, was lifting a heavy bed up a flight of stairs he developed lower back pain that radiated down his left leg. He had also noticed some numbness in his left leg.

Barry tried painkillers, physiotherapy and acupuncture, but endured a further six months of severe pain before visiting my clinic. Barry was no longer going to the gym due to his pain. An MRI scan of Barry's lower back showed a disc prolapse that was pressing on his nerve root supplying his left leg. I gave Barry a steroid injection into his lower back, and after a month, the symptoms in his lower back and left leg had subsided. Barry worked in a sedentary job, sitting most days, hence his lower back structures were not as strong as those of someone performing manual labour such as a furniture remover. Ensuring you have adequate help when lifting very heavy furniture may avoid injury.

are wedge-shaped to create this curve.

If the vertebrae and discs were square then the spine would be straight, but problems would arise at the bottom of the spine due to the pressure generated. The weight of each vertebra would add to the pressure, resulting in the bottom of the column collapsing.

The beauty of the spinal column's design is in the way it absorbs forces. If you load the spine by placing a heavy container on your head or shoulders, the curve increases, reducing the height of the column. On unloading the heavy object, the spine would stretch again. Instead of crushing the bottom of the spine, pressure is relieved at the middle of the curve. It is essentially acting as a C-shaped spring that compresses when the spine is loaded and unwinds when the load is removed.

If a disc in the lower back is causing pain, it is best to reduce pressure on that disc. This will cause less electricity to flow from the disc through to the brain, reducing pain. It pays to think about activities and modify the way you perform them.

When the back is in its normal curved shape, the pressure on the discs and the bones is at a minimum. However, if the curve is straightened by postures such as leaning forward for prolonged periods, pressure is placed on the discs that can lead to disc compression and pain.

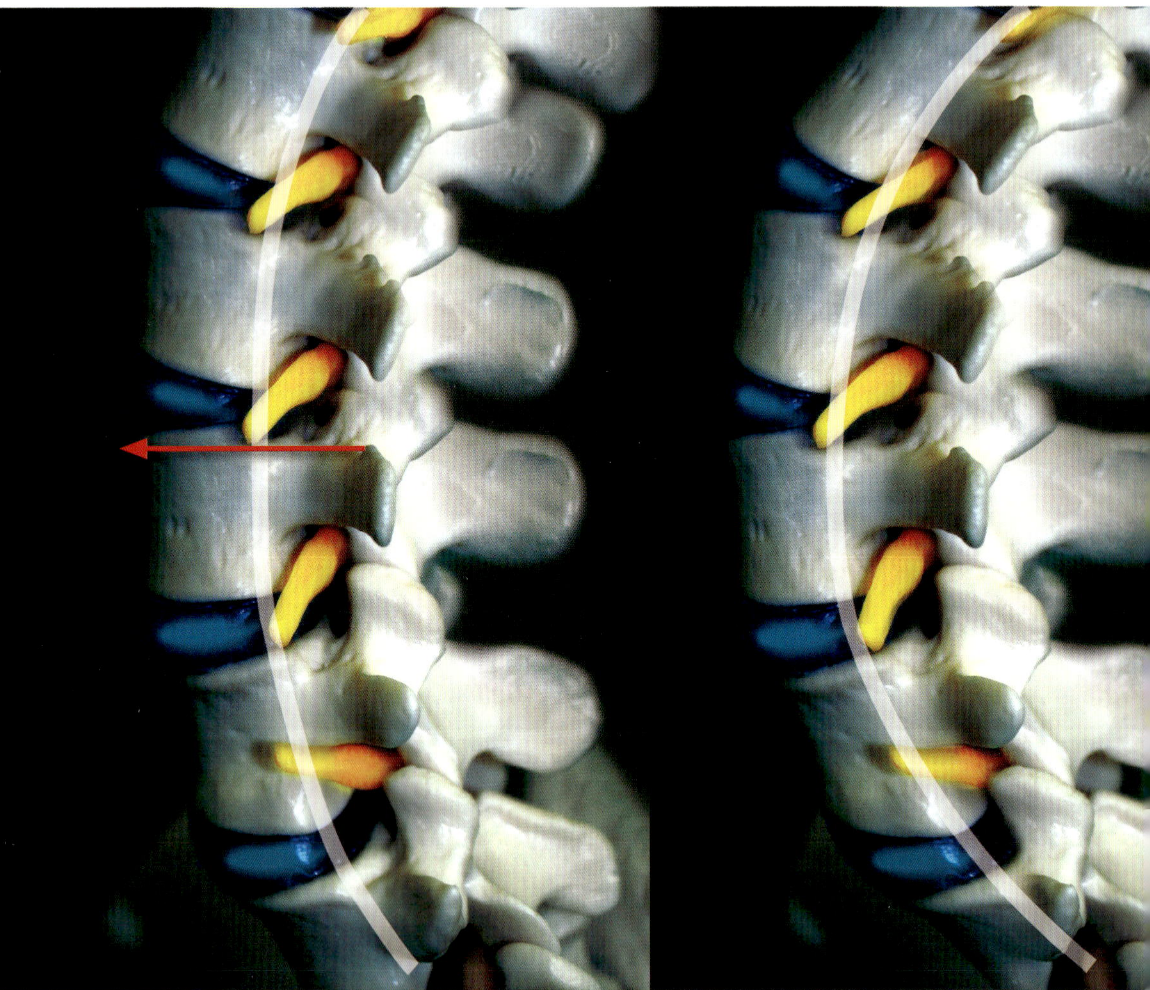

Figure 5.1

The lower back has a C-shaped curve. The curve increases on loading the lower back as shown on the right-hand side.

Figure 5.2

When the normal curve of the lower back is lost, as shown on the right-hand side, pressure is exerted on the lowest disc. The arrows indicate the direction of pressure acting on the spine.

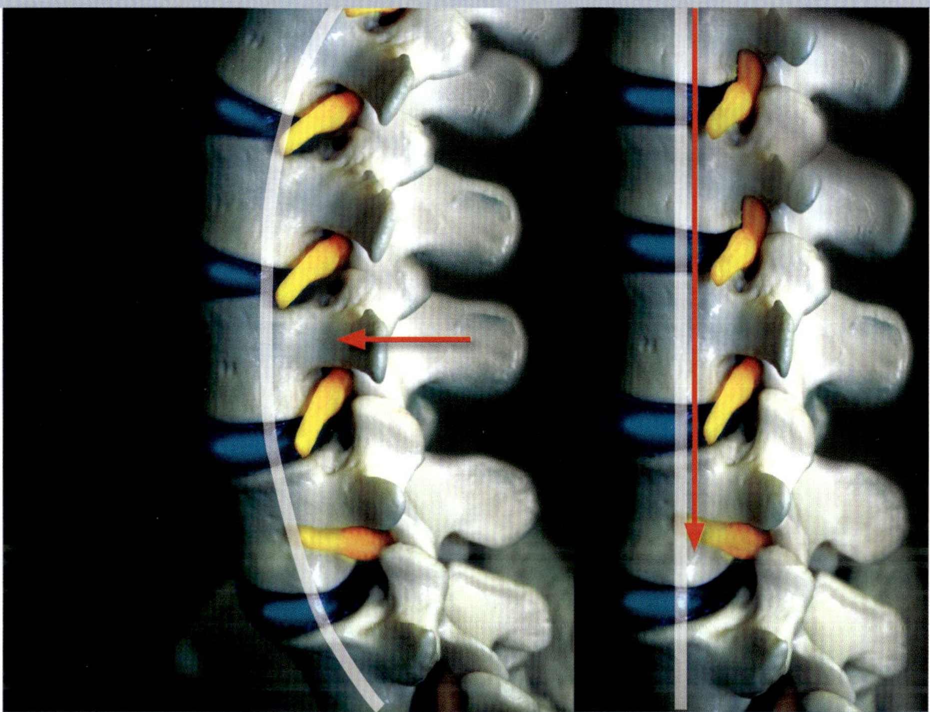

3. Maintain good sitting posture

Sitting for long periods of time places gravitational pressure through the spine, resulting in pressure on the lower back discs that will build up with time. People can sit for variable periods before experiencing lower back pain. If you have lower back pain, it is advisable to get up and down frequently to avoid pressure building up with time. Sometimes a reminder can be helpful. There are many basic computer programs available that prompt desk-bound workers to get out of their chairs at regular intervals.

When you are sitting, always try and maintain your lower back curve, as shown in *Figure 5.3*. Remember this is the natural shape of the lower back and will cause the least amount of pressure on the discs of the lower back. Sitting or leaning forward increases the pressure on the lower back discs, often causing pain. A lumbar roll can be helpful in maintaining this curve, as shown in *Figure 5.4*. Most chair manufacturers make chairs with a curve in the back, so sit against the back of the chair and don't lean forward. Sitting against the back of the chair also ensures that some of your weight is transferred through the back of the chair instead of compressing your lower back.

Making a habit of leaning to one side when sitting as shown in *Figure 5.5* will result in pressure on one side of the discs in the lower back that may cause

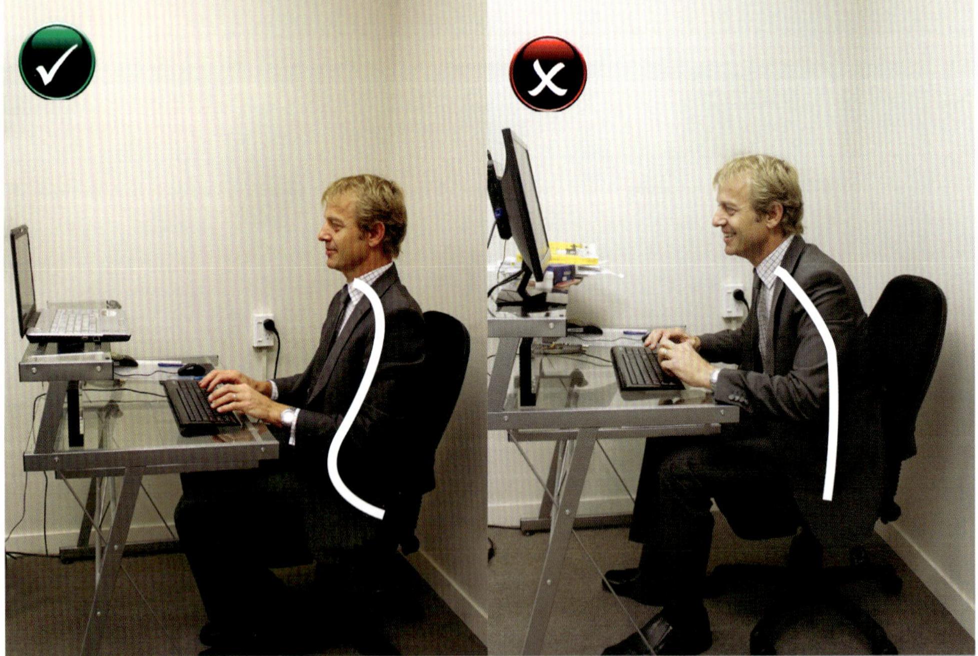

Figure 5.3

The left-hand picture shows a good sitting posture, with a curve in the lower back. The posture on the right straightens the curve and increases the pressure on the lowest discs in the lower back.

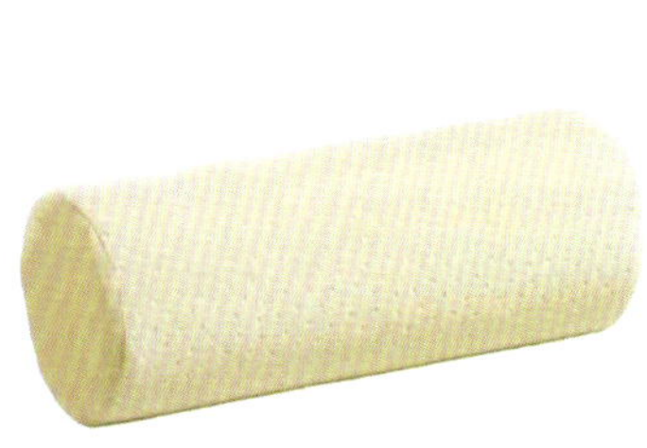

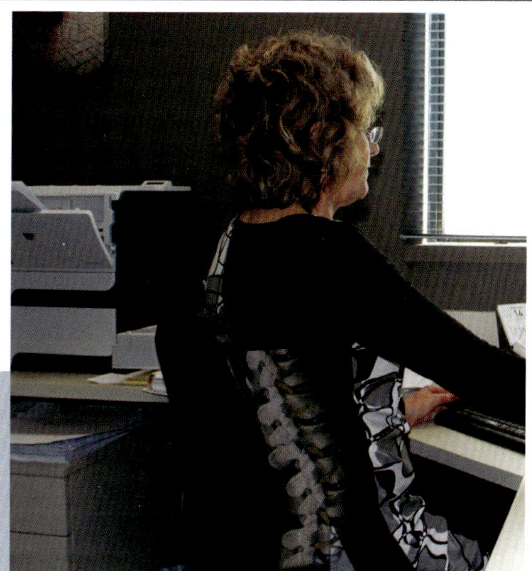

Figure 5.4
The lumbar roll shown above helps to maintain the curve in the lower back while sitting.

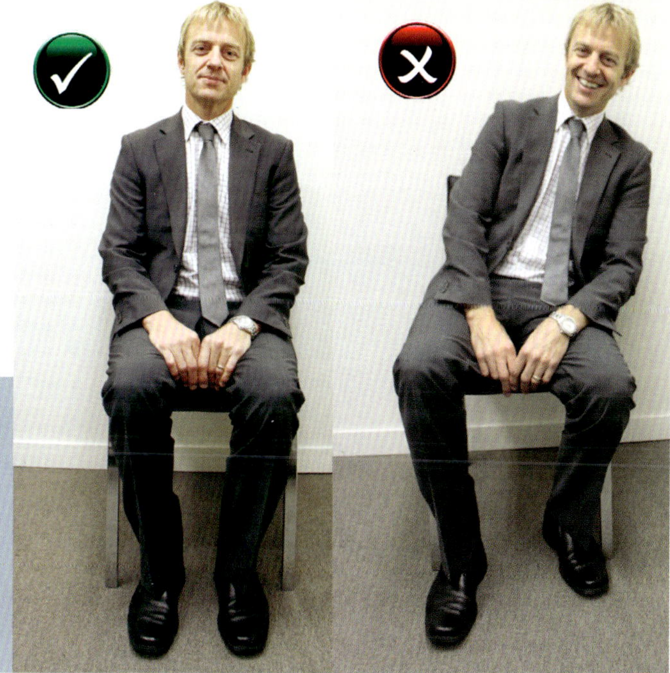

Figure 5.5
When sitting, sit without a lean, as shown on the left-hand picture. Sitting with a lean places excessive pressure on one side of the discs in the lower back.

deterioration of the ring ligament.

One way to reduce gravitational pressure is to sit on a recliner chair, as the pressure passes through the chair rather than compressing the spine. This will reduce pressure on the lower back discs, reducing pain. Recliner chairs vary and, to ensure you obtain the right fit, always sit on the recliner in the shop for 20 to 30 minutes before purchasing it.

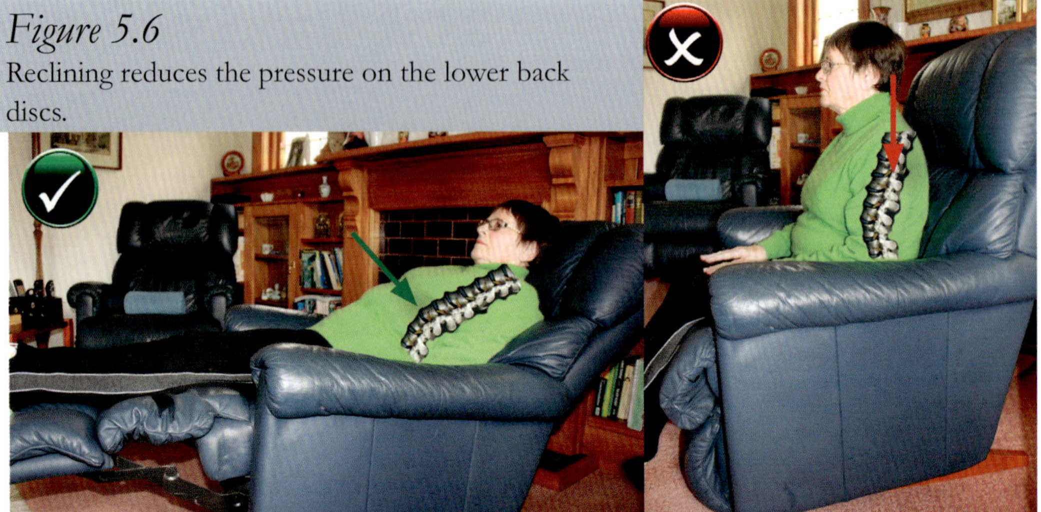

Figure 5.6
Reclining reduces the pressure on the lower back discs.

4. Maintain good bending posture

Activities that require you to bend forward place enormous pressure on the discs of the lower back. Not only is the curve of the lower back lost, but the pressure from the trunk increases two to three times due to the angles created. Vacuuming, ironing, leaning over the kitchen sink and gardening are activities that require leaning forward.

When standing at the sink, bend your knees, and place one leg in front of the other to help maintain the curve in your lower back, as shown in *Figure 5.7*. Try this position with one leg forward and then the other, as people often find one of these positions more comfortable. If you stand with your legs together and bend forward, the pressure on the lower back discs multiplies many times. When vacuuming, ensure the pipe is extended to minimise forward bending, as shown in *Figure 5.8*. When gardening, sitting may reduce the pressure on the lower back compared to bending as shown in *Figure 5.9*.

Figure 5.7

Standing with your knees bent with one leg in front of the other over the sink or bench, rather than with both legs together, will reduce the pressure on the discs in the lower back.

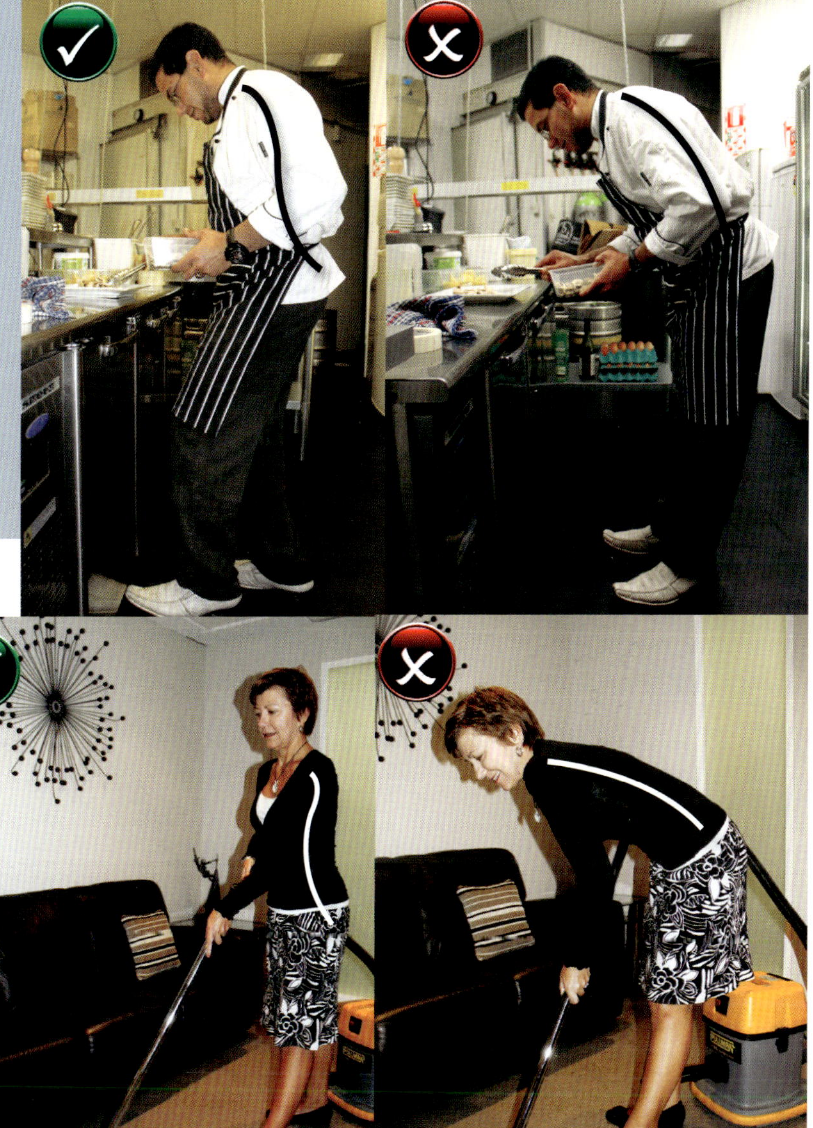

Figure 5.8

In the left-hand photo vacuuming with an extended pipe creates less pressure on the lower back. In the right-hand photo, when vacuuming with a short pipe, increased bending is required that places pressure on the lower back discs.

Figure 5.9
Gardening with a bent back and straight legs increases the pressure on lower back discs several-fold. Gardening in new positions, such as sitting down, may help reduce pain.

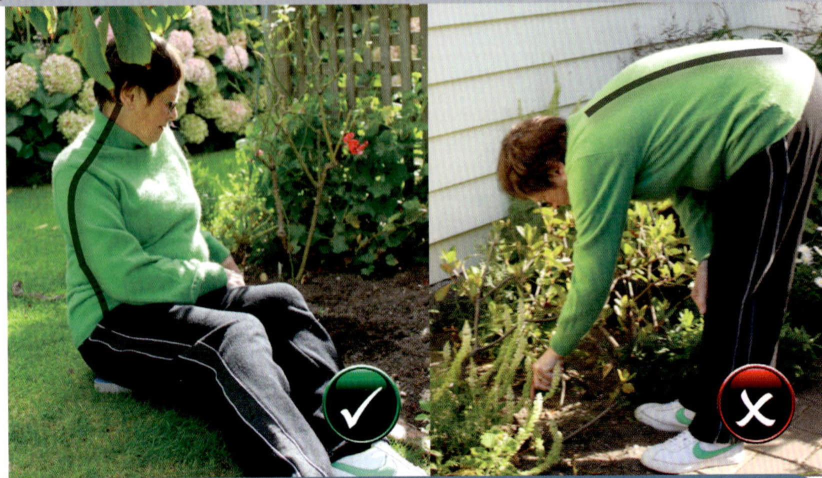

5. Lift with good technique

When lifting, always hold the object close to your body, as this reduces the pressure exerted on the lower back discs *(Figure 5.10)*. Bending your knees

Figure 5.10
The pressure exerted on the lower back discs is significantly less when you hold the load you are lifting close to your body.

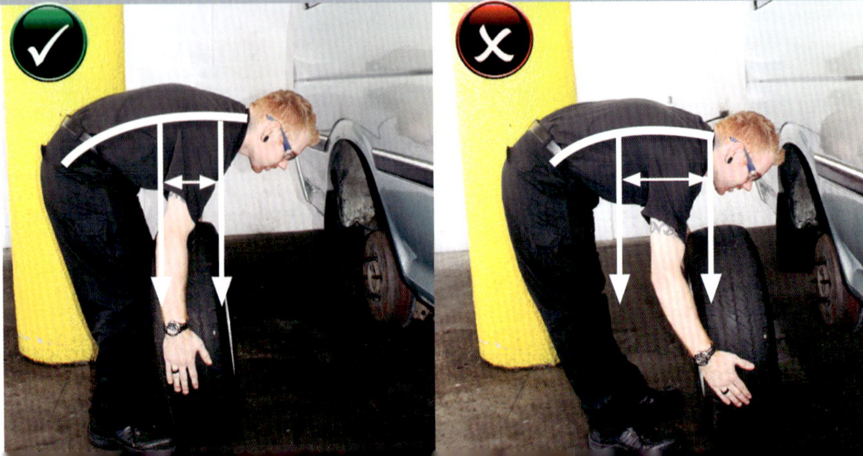

while lifting helps maintain the curve in your lower back and reduces the pressure on the lower back discs *(Figure 5.11)*.

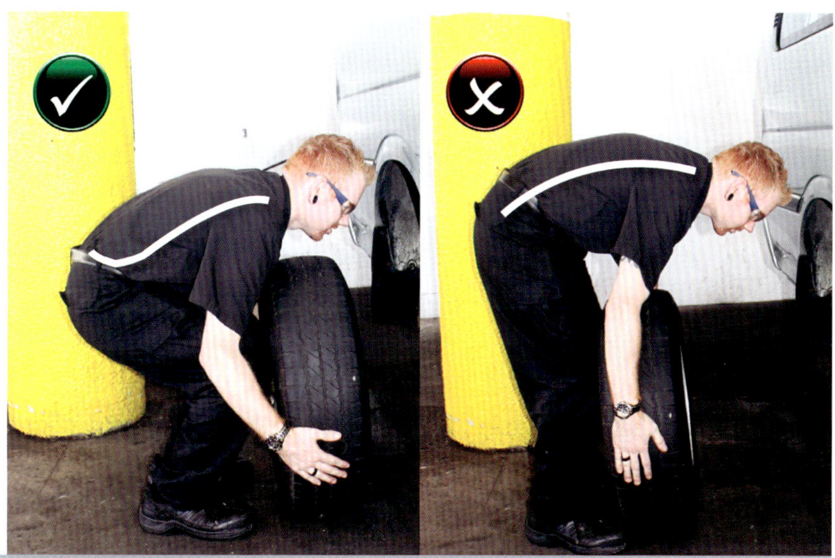

Figure 5.11
Bending your knees when preparing to lift an object helps to maintain the curve of your spine when lifting.

6. Try inversion therapy (stretch your back)

The disc is the most common source of pain in the lower back and just as pressure on the disc creates pain, distracting the disc can often help pain. Using gravity to stretch the disc will encourage fluid to return it, alleviating pressure on the top and bottom of the disc. You may have seen many contraptions designed to suspend you upside down as shown in *Figure 5.12*. Lying suspended at 30 to 40 degrees for three to five minutes twice a day may reduce the number of painkillers required and is one way of managing the pain at its source. If the pain is not stemming from the disc then this may not help the pain.

In 1964, a study of 175 people[4] with lower back pain who were off work showed that 155 returned to work with inversion. Studies have shown that inversion relaxes the muscles in the lower back. In 2012, a study of people with disc prolapse[5] demonstrated how useful inversion can be. Of the inversion group, 2/10 required an operation, whereas in the other group without inversion 8/10 of the patients required an operation. If pain arises from the discs then inversion is likely to help.

Some people cannot tolerate lying upside down and affordability may be a problem. There are some simple stretches that also distract the low back discs. One way is to suspend the body to exert a pull on the lower back discs is to lie on the bed, on your front, with some of the chest off the bed and let yourself hang for five minutes, two to three times a day. Several patients who could not perform inversion have been advised to perform this simple exercise for five minutes several times a day with good improvements in their lower back pain. This simple stretch is shown in *Figure 5.13*. The stretch shown in *Figure 5.14* also stretches the low back disc and should be performed for a few minutes two or three times a day.

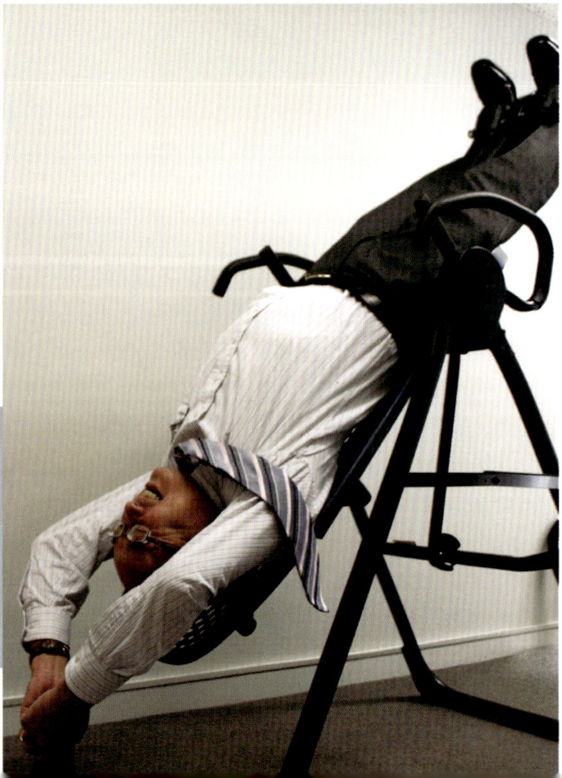

Figure 5.12

Inversion machines are designed to suspend people upside down to relieve pressure within the lower back discs.

Figure 5.13

Lying on the bed with part of the upper body off the bed can also exert a stretch on the lower back.

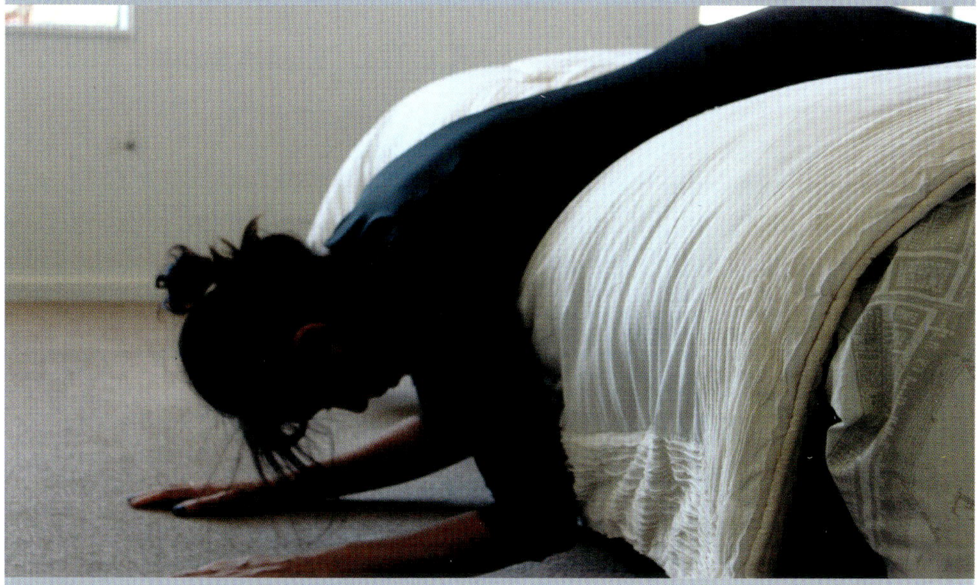

Figure 5.14

Lying on your back with your knees bent holding them also stretches the lower back.

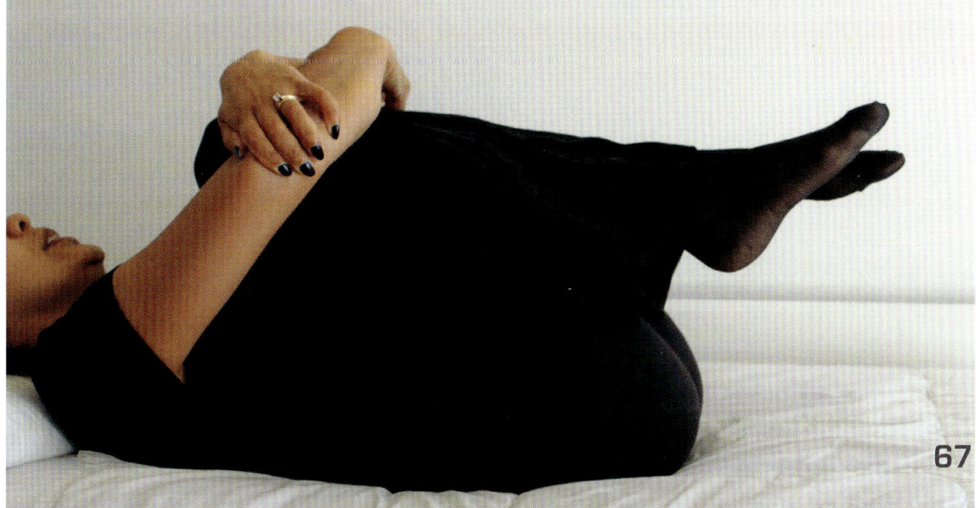

CASE STUDY: *Germon*

Forty-six-year-old *Germon* was at the gym performing leg presses with heavy weights when he slipped and twisted his lower back. He developed lower back pain that spread into his groin and inner thigh. He thought he had strained a muscle and continued attending the gym and tried stretching, but the pain continued to worsen.

After a month, Germon started waking at three a.m. with excruciating pain in his groin and inner thigh region and could not return to sleep. During the day, the pain was okay and he managed to work in his office position and perform most other activities, including playing golf.

Germon's symptoms continued for six months. An MRI scan of his lower back showed significant disc narrowing and a bright signal in the adjacent bones, as seen overleaf. A bright signal is caused when a disc fails to absorb pressure, placing increased pressure on the surrounding bone, causing fluid to build up in the adjacent bone. It is likely that the disc narrowing and dehydration of the discs were present before the recent accident but the factor causing his pain was the adjacent bones. Germon was involved in a high impact motor vehicle accident as a child and this may have been the original initiating factor in the deterioration of his lower back discs.

Germon continued to attend the gym but adapted his activities to avoid pressure on the discs of the lower back. He stopped performing weights sitting and started more bar exercises. His groin pain settled but he continued to experience lower back pain. He bought a new memory foam mattress for his bed and immediately started to sleep until six a.m. He also started using an inversion machine on a daily basis, which helped his symptoms.

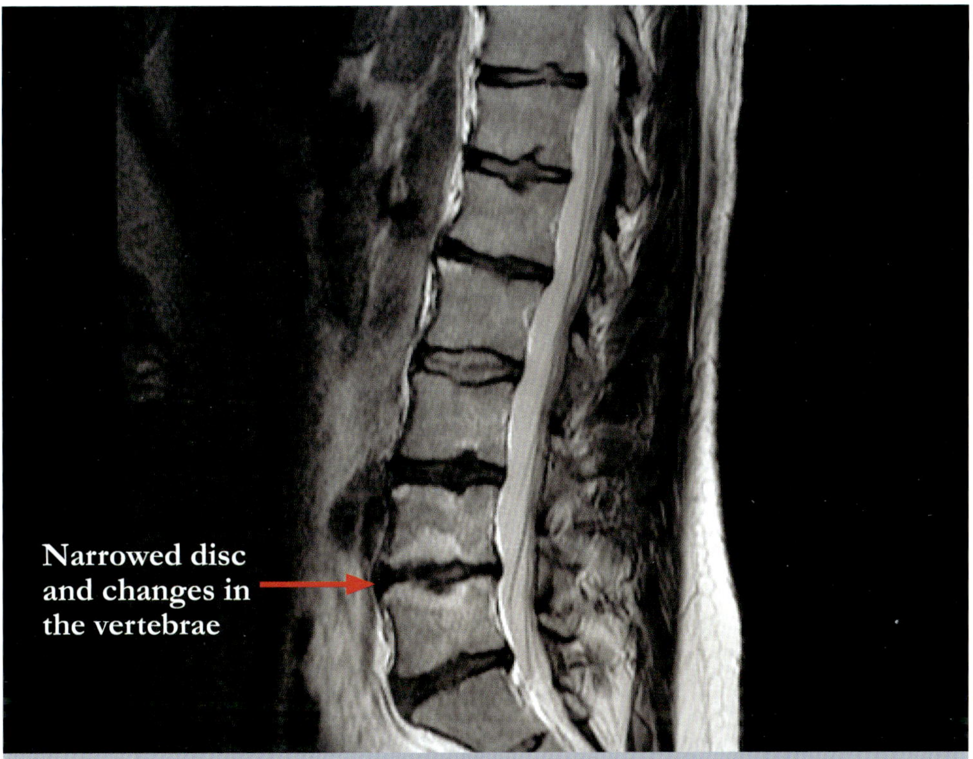

Figure 5.15 *Germon's* MRI scan shows a narrowed disc and adjacent bright signals representing bony stress.

7. Ensure good sleeping posture

Many people experience lower back pain while sleeping or wake with pain and stiffness. The pain emanates from the lower back due to the position that the lower back adopts in the bed. When sleeping on the side of the body, the shoulder hits the bed and the hip hits the bed. The lower back, however, often bends which creates pressure building up in one side of the discs, as shown in *Figure 5.16*. This pressure creates electrical sparks which travel to the brain, resulting in pain. The electrical sparks build with time, hence the pain increases with time and, often, after a few hours you wake with pain. As described in the case of Germon, sometimes you cannot get back to sleep after being woken.

Commonly, painkillers or tablets that cause sedation are prescribed to reduce sleep disturbance. Painkillers and sedative tablets suppress electrical signals in the brain however the electrical sparks are produced in the lower back, usually due to pressure. Obviously, it would be better to suppress the pain at

Figure 5.16

The top figure shows a straight spine while sleeping on one's side which maintains the least pressure on the lower back discs. The curved spine in the bottom figure shows poor sleeping posture leading to increased disc pressure, often leading to pain at night.

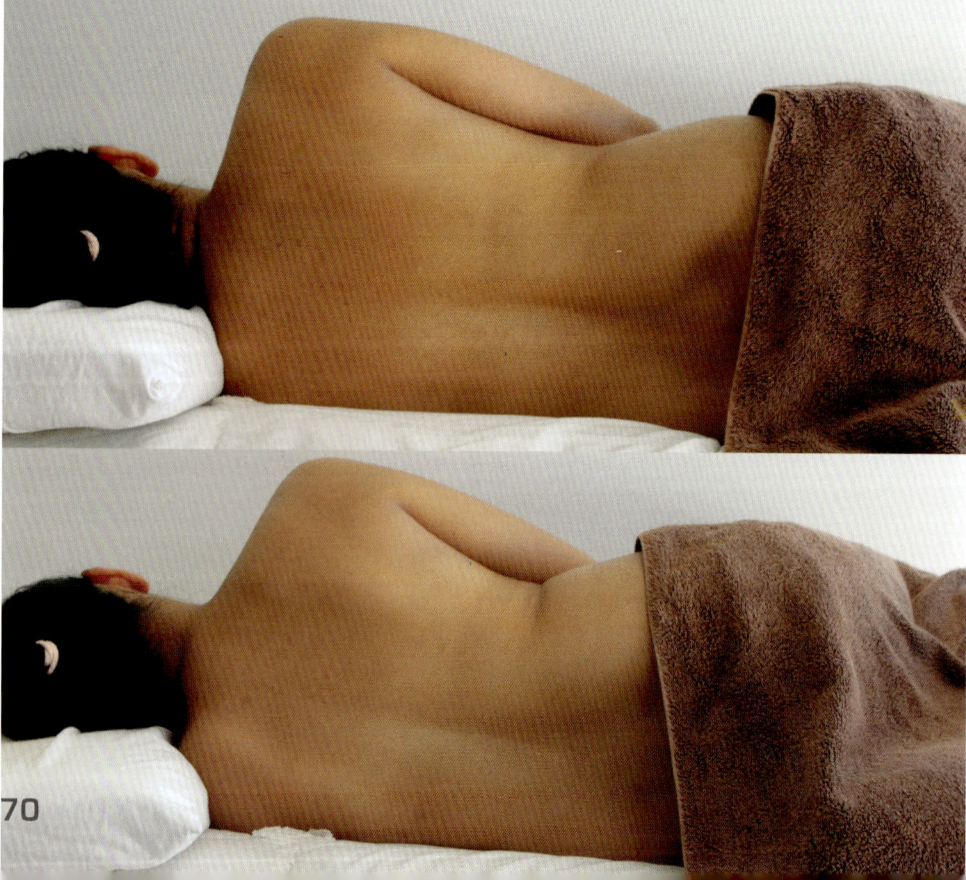

the level of the lower back discs to improve sleep.

If sleep is disturbed at night, changing the position of the spine by trying different mattresses can be helpful. A memory foam mattress is substantially different from an innersprung mattress and creates a different pressure profile which can help some patients with their night pain. Essentially, the shoulder and hip that hit the bed sink into the bed when sleeping on your side. This creates support to the spine which reduces the curve and hence reduces pressure on the discs.

To improve sleep disturbance from lower back pain, some patients have tried another bed in the house and found they wake less at night. Many patients have arranged a trial of the new bed or mattress to see if this helps pain. Remember to try and arrange a trial of a new bed or mattress that you can return if the new bed does not help improve sleep. Unfortunately, I hear too often of how people have spent plenty of money buying a new bed only to find it has not helped their symptoms and they cannot return it.

8. Maintain core strength

Many people treating lower back pain will give advice on improving core strength. Core strength can be described as a balloon of muscles that surrounds the lower back (*Figure 5.17*) and supports the spine whenever we perform activities such as walking, bending and lifting.

Pain switches off the core muscles, which in turn increases movement and pressure on the discs at the base of the spine causing pain. If activity becomes painful, people stop activity, further compromising their core strength. Unfortunately, a cycle is set up whereby increased pain leads to reduced activity, weakening the core further and making activity even more difficult.

Keep fit and perform physical activity at least four times a week for 30 to 60 minutes. It does not matter what form of exercise you choose as long as it gets the heart racing and the body moving. This will maintain good core strength and prevent future recurrences of back pain, especially for pain arising from the discs.

When returning to activity, choose exercise that does not aggravate pain. If exercise increases lower back pain, then it is likely to be placing pressure on the lower back discs and hence stimulating pain. Sometimes it is difficult to advise exactly which activity is the most suitable, as different people may have disc damage at different levels and different activities may cause pain for each individual. Trial and error is the best approach. Try cycling, swimming, walking or using a cross trainer and see how long you can perform the activity without significant pain. Aquajogging, using a flotation belt in the pool, is the activity least likely to aggravate pain. The water suspends your weight and reduces the pressure placed on the disc.

Figure 5.17

The core is like a balloon of muscles that supports the lower back. The right-hand diagram shows a reduced core strength resulting in increased movement of the lower spine.

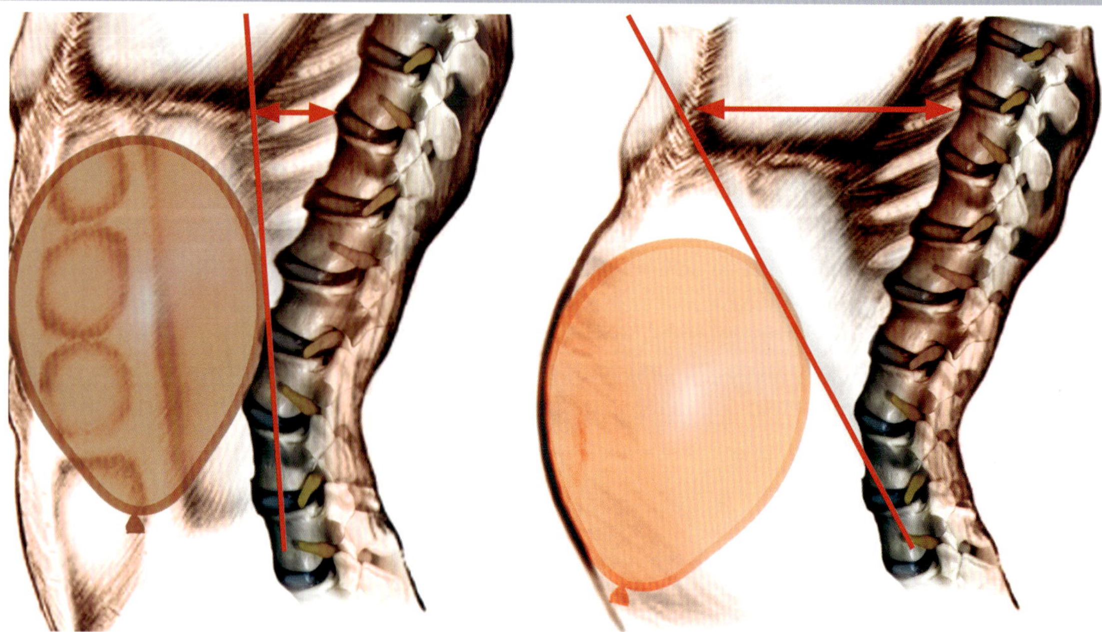

Core strength is only one of several factors that influences lower back pain. The extent of disc damage, pressure placed on the discs by activities and your pain threshold are also important determinants of lower back pain. For many people who already have a good level of fitness, increasing core strength is unlikely to improve their lower back pain.

CASE STUDY: *Natasha*

Natasha regularly competed in triathlons and tended to develop lower back pain on the last leg of these races. She recalled a bad episode of back pain 20 years before presenting when she fell playing netball as a student. The MRI scan of her lower back seen below showed a narrowed disc with stress on the adjacent bones. This damage had been sustained 20 years previously and the disc had narrowed slowly until it was no longer able to absorb pressure, increasing the pressure on the adjacent bones.

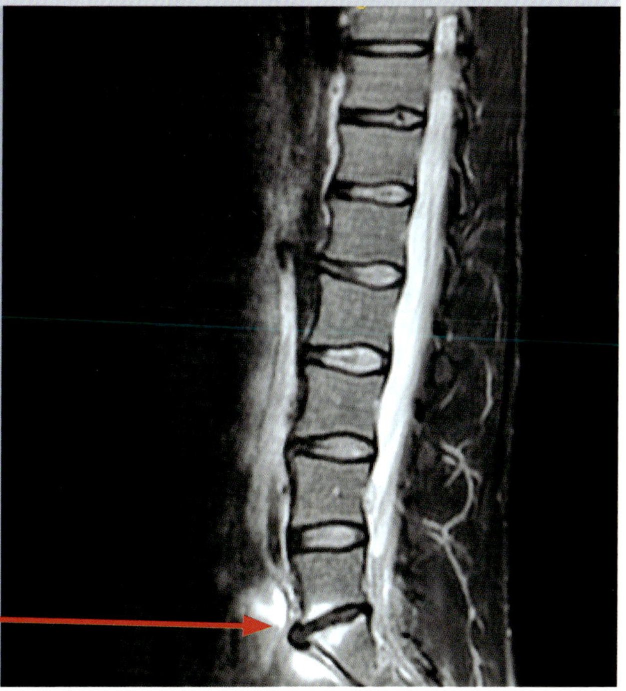

Figure 5.18

The MRI scan shows narrowing of the lowest disc in the lower back as well as a loss of hydration in the disc. The scan also shows a reduction in the curve of the lower back. The whitening along the edges of the bone adjacent to the damaged disc shows increased fluid, which is a sign of bony stress.

Narrowing disc with bony stress surrounding disc (shown in white).

CASE STUDY: *Elizabeth*

70-year-old *Elizabeth* had a large sideways curve of her spine, as shown on the right-hand image below. She had a hip replacement due to arthritis of the hip and stopped her regular pool-based exercises for six weeks while she recovered. She noticed an increase in her lower back pain. Her pain increased for two reasons: first, the reduced exercise caused a loss of core strength; second, she had been used to walking with a limp, shifting her weight to one side of her body. Following her hip replacement, she started walking straighter and placing more pressure on the spinal discs causing pain. In returning to her pool-based exercises and with time, Elizabeth's symptoms subsided as her back adjusted to her new posture.

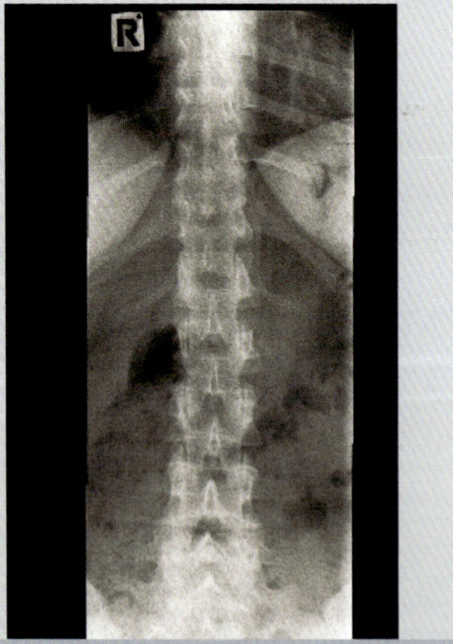

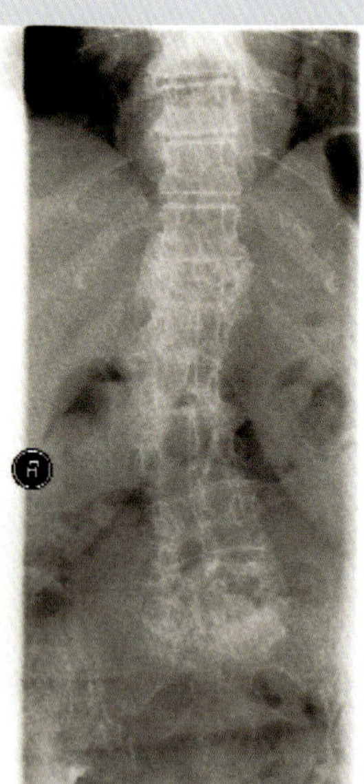

Figure 5.19

The X-ray on the left shows the normal shape of the spine looking from the front, which is straight. The X-ray on the right shows a marked curve of the spine when looking straight-on. This is referred to as a scoliosis.

Improving core strength by performing simple activities that do not cause pain is the best approach. A simple sit-up with knees bent, placing the hands on the stomach and only raising the shoulders slightly off the bed is a good option. Hold the position for five seconds and repeat ten times morning and night. The picture below (*Figure 5.20*) shows the initial and final position to be held for five seconds. When you perform this simple sit-up you can feel the stomach muscles contract against your hands.

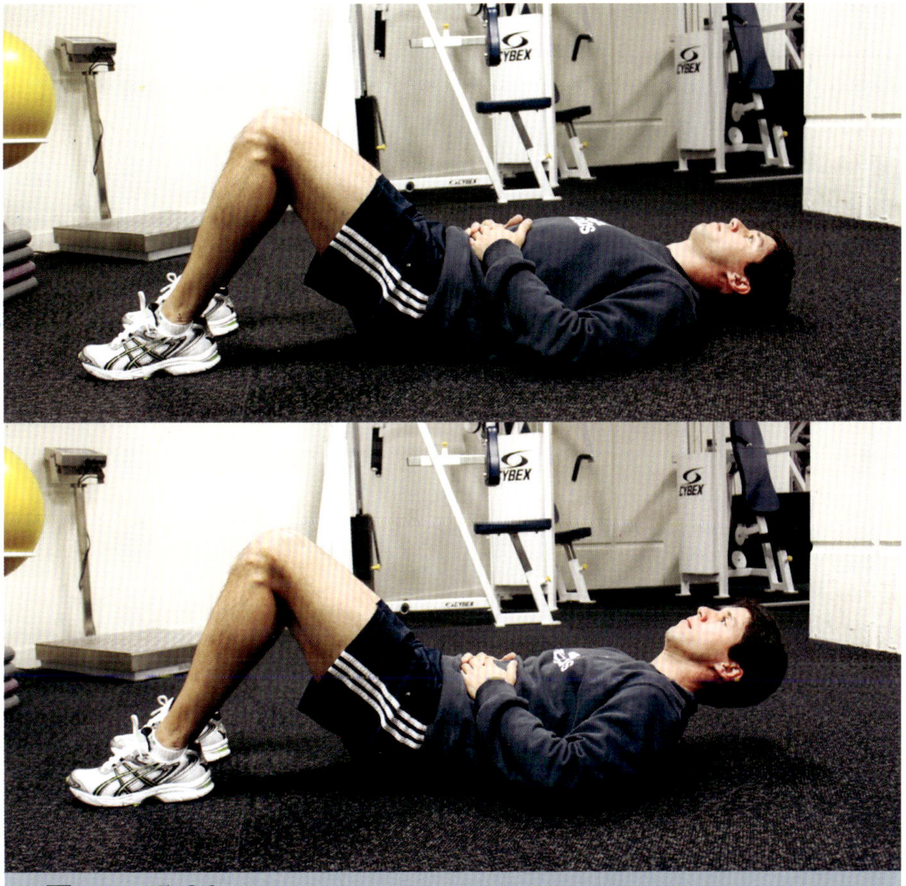

Figure 5.20

The top photo shows the start position for this sit-up, and the bottom photo shows the final position.

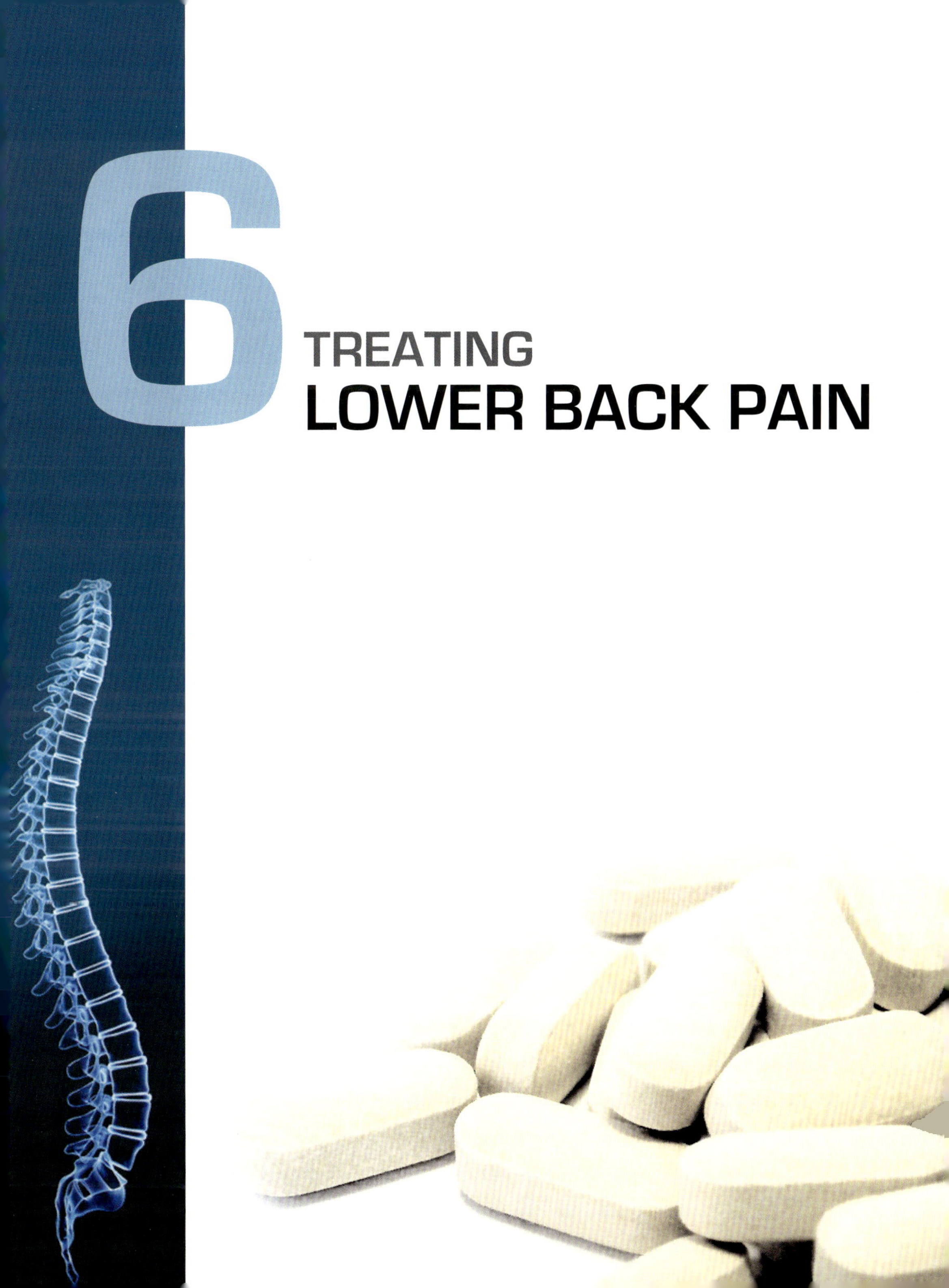

6 TREATING LOWER BACK PAIN

What do you do if your lower back pain is not improving? There are many treatments available for back pain and countless promises of miracle cures. This chapter will outline some of the pharmaceutical options and commonly available hands-on treatments for lower back pain.

In clinical trials of painkillers, different medications are tested against chalk tablets (placebo) to see if they yield better results. Most vitamins, minerals and natural therapies are not tested to see if they are better than placebo, making them less-tested remedies.

What does the research show about the effectiveness of different treatment approaches? Most clinical trials show that attending a therapist for lower back pain is not very effective when you have long-term lower back pain. A pragmatic approach is to start with simple treatments and progress to more invasive or unpleasant management options. It is also useful if the therapy can be performed at home, saving time and money, including traveling to appointments, time off work and the money required to pay health professionals' fees.

The disc is the most likely source of pain in the lower back. Hence, treatment aimed at the disc is best tried first. In the last year, as the affordability of inversion machines has improved, many patients have bought their own machines and suspend themselves two or three times a day for a few minutes. Not only does this reduce disc pressure, it also relaxes the surrounding muscles. The majority of patients using this approach have noticed a marked improvement in their symptoms, often over four to six weeks. If an affordable machine can be sourced, then this is certainly the best initial approach for lower back pain.

If inversion therapy does not help, then it may be worth trying various treatment options for six to eight sessions. If there is improvement, stick with the provider, otherwise change to another treatment approach.

Some treatments are aimed at the muscle, such as massage, acupuncture or stretching. Others, such as mobilisation or manipulation, are directed at the joints of the lower back. Sometimes, pain may improve for a short period, only to return later. Often, the painful muscle or tight joint is not the source of the pain, but instead an underlying disc is the source which spreads pain into the muscles and causes joint tightness.

Medications

You may recall from Chapter 2 that pain is due to electrical signals travelling in nerves to the brain. On the whole, medications that relieve pain act at the brain to reduce electricity and hence diminish pain, as shown in *Figure 6.1*. Medications do not generally act at the site of pain. In the case of the lower back discs, the electrical spark produced is in response to pressure. Controlling pain by altering the pressure on the discs through inversion and changing the way you perform activity is preferable. However, medications may help when pain is severe or you are waiting for improvement from treatment.

Several types of medication are prescribed for lower back pain, ranging from anti-inflammatories to tablets used for epilepsy and depression. Often patients go to the pharmacy to collect their medication to discover, to their horror, that they have been prescribed an antidepressant.

It is important to remember that there is no one tablet for all. Individuals often respond differently to different tablets, so what helps one person may not help another. Furthermore, one person may develop side effects while another develops no side effects. It is a case of trial and error most of the time, so if a tablet is not helping or causing side effects, then go back to the doctor and try another.

The medications commonly prescribed for lower back pain are paracetamol, anti-inflammatories, opiates and tramadol. Combinations of medications are also commonly prescribed or can be purchased over the counter. Paracetamol works on the brain pain pathways and is the first line painkiller for muscle and joint pain due to its minimal side effects. The standard paracetamol tablet gives pain relief for approximately four hours. The main side effect of paracetamol is liver toxicity when given in overdose.

Non-steroidal anti-inflammatory drugs include aspirin, ibuprofen, diclofenac, naproxen, meloxicam, and many others. In up to 15 percent of people taking these

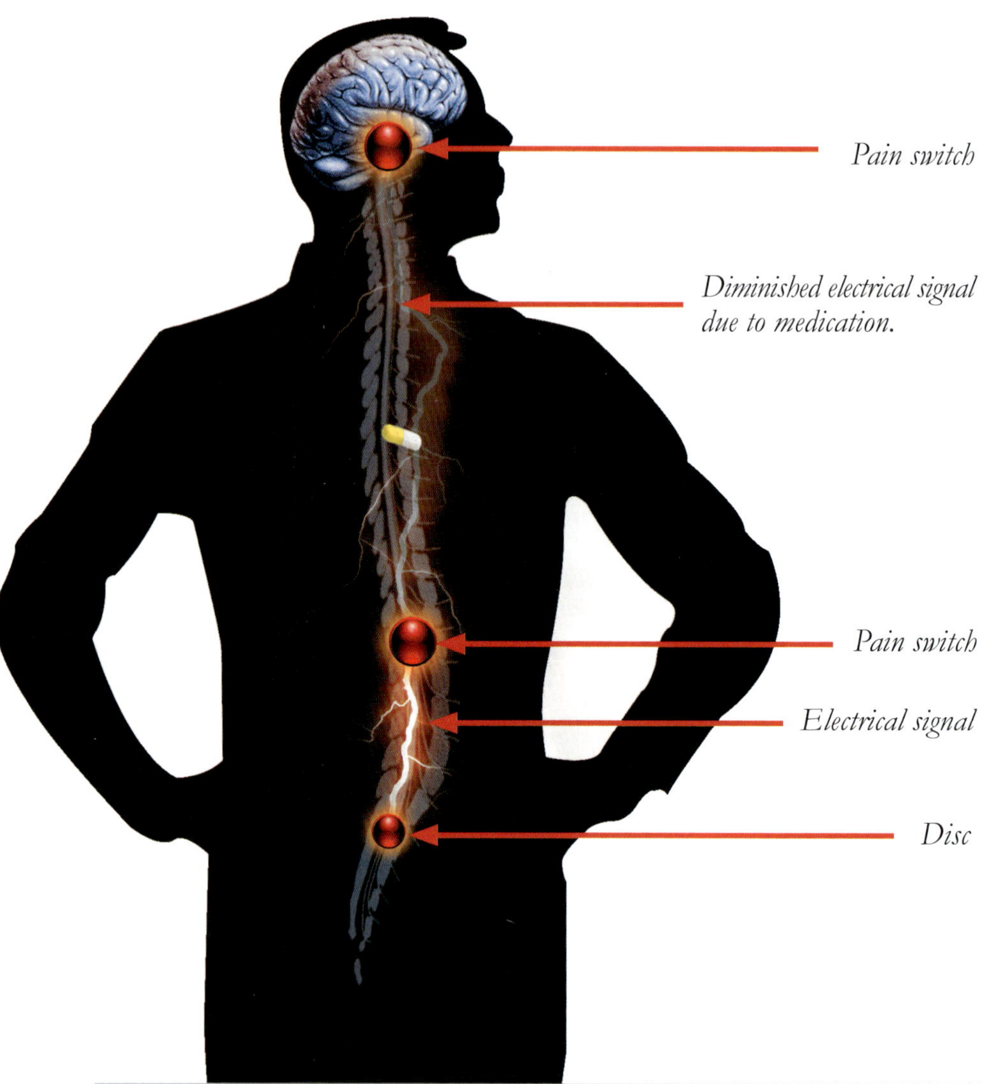

Figure 6.1

Medications reduce the electricity that conducts pain in the brain rather than act at the source of the pain.

drugs, gastric bleeding occurs and can lead to stomach ulcers. If abdominal discomfort occurs, you should stop these tablets and see your doctor. These drugs can increase asthma symptoms as well as cause kidney and liver damxage, usually with long-term usage.

The commonly prescribed opiate medications are codeine, morphine, pethidine and methadone. Tramadol is an opiate-like medication. Codeine is usually the first-line opiate medication and, while effective for most people, ten percent of people cannot turn it into the active ingredient once swallowed. It is available over the counter combined with both paracetamol and ibuprofen. Taken in combination, it is thought to be slightly more effective. Codeine can cause drowsiness, which may be helpful at night if sleep is disturbed. Constipation can also be a problem if codeine is taken regularly. Stronger opiates, including pethidine and morphine, are also available on prescription. All opiates are addictive if taken regularly and for prolonged periods. If they are taken long-term, patients often need to withdraw gradually rather than stop abruptly.

Several medications such as orphenadrine (Norflex) and diazepam are prescribed to reduce muscle spasm. Orphenadrine is an antihistamine and is often found in cold medications. Diazepam is better known as Valium and is a sleeping tablet that is addictive.

Certain antidepressants such as amitriptyline and nortriptyline are prescribed in low doses for lower back pain. They are useful to help the patient sleep and may dull the pain a little as well. These tablets act on many receptors and have many side effects. Unfortunately, the elderly can experience dizziness, dry mouth and daytime sedation from these tablets. Antipsychotics can also be prescribed in low doses to reduce pain by improving sleep.

Medications for lower back pain are a useful adjunct to management best used for acute bouts of severe pain rather than regularly. Many medications lose their effectiveness when taken regularly, as the brain becomes familar with the medication and responds less. This tolerance leads to patients requiring escalating doses of medications to achieve the same effect. This is especially true for opiates.

Manual therapy

Manual therapy is any therapy that is performed by hand. For lower back pain, this usually includes massage, mobilisation and manipulation. People with lower back pain often experience muscle tightness and spasm. A cycle often develops whereby a deeper structure is damaged such as the disc, which in turn creates muscle spasm and subsequent joint tightness, leaving someone with a feeling of stiffness. A combination of treating the muscles together with mobilisation or manipulation of the joints may relieve the feeling of tightness.

Massage

Massage therapy can be gentle for relaxation or rigorous and stimulate pain. Massage therapy often heats the area and increases blood flow. There is also a feedback mechanism to the pain centres of the muscle, spinal cord and brain when the skin is massaged. People find massage useful for relief of symptoms. If pain is caused by muscles, then massage has the potential to relieve pain totally, such as for a muscle strain. However, if the pain is stemming from a deeper structure such as the disc, joint or bone, massage may offer short-term alleviation but is unlikely to resolve the problem long-term.

Mobilisation

Mobilisation is like manipulation (cracking of the joints), but is performed with less vigour and no sudden forces. The joint is slowly moved and stretched. It is gentler than manipulation and achieves similar results. Therapists are often trained to both mobilise and manipulate joints and use these techniques on a case-by-case basis.

Manipulation

Manipulation of joints is a sudden, vigorous movement used classically by chiropractors to improve spinal pain. It is an ancient art of healing, and many people swear by its effectiveness to relieve symptoms in their neck and back. *Figure 6.2* shows the classic back manipulation sometimes called the 'million dollar roll' due to the money it generates for practitioners.

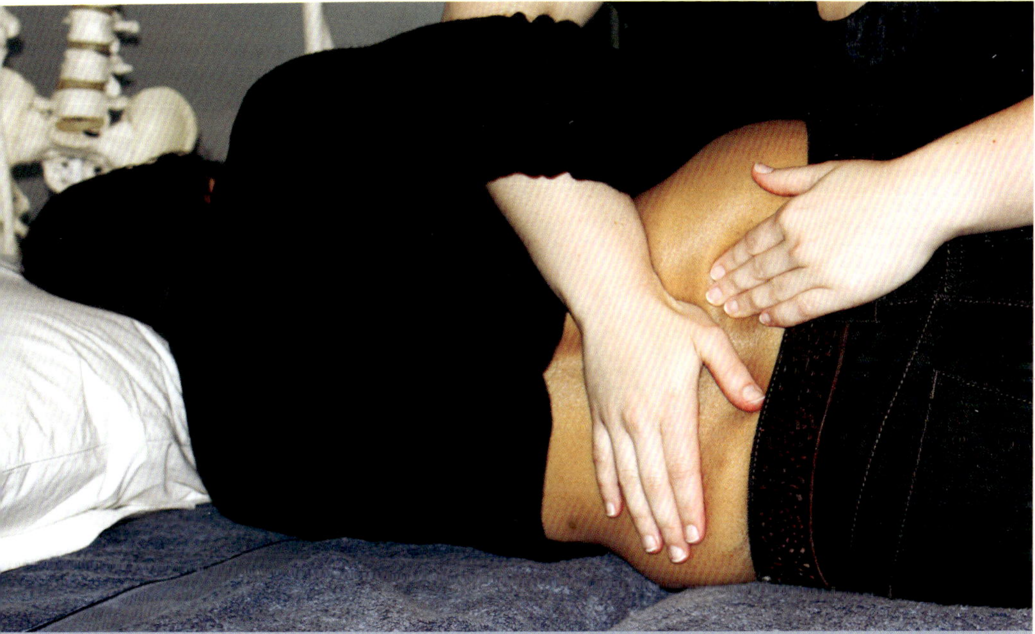

Figure 6.2
Manipulation of the lower back.

Needle therapies

Needle therapies for back pain include acupuncture, muscle needling and injections of solutions into the soft tissues.

Acupuncture

In acupuncture, a thin needle is inserted into soft tissues such as the skin, muscle, tendon or ligament (*Figure 6.3*). The needle is often inserted into the most tender area and produces a dull aching sensation. It is very safe, and bleeding is often minimal, as the needle is fine and cannot easily pierce blood vessels.

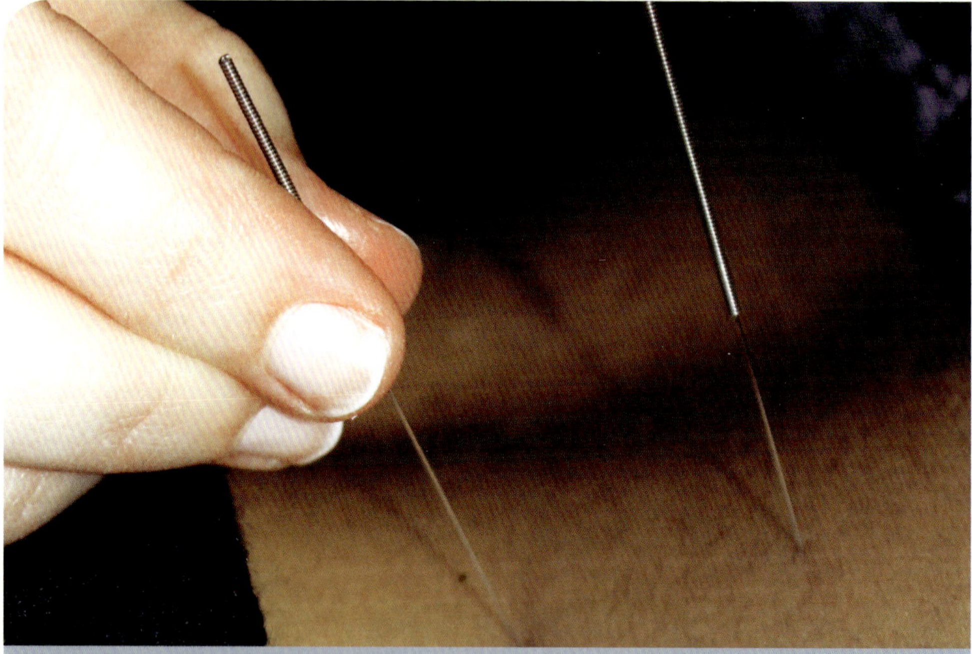

Figure 6.3
An acupuncture needle being inserted into the skin and muscle.

Injections

Several injection therapies have been promoted for lower back pain, including botox, prolotherapy (injecting an irritant to stimulate healing) and anaesthetic injections. In studies of lower back pain, salt water (saline) injections have been found to be just as effective as prolotherapy and botox. This may be due to either the insertion of the needle or the injected solution washing away the chemicals that cause electricity in the pain switches of the muscles.

When a large study[5] showed that prolotherapy and saline injections gave similar improvements for lower back pain, I started injecting saline into painful areas because it is cheap, effective and has no side effects. In 2006, I treated 100 consecutive patients with long-term back pain (pain present for an average of six years) with saline injections[6]. I injected with saline the lower back ligaments, muscles and tendons that were tender. Of these patients 34 had 100 percent improvement in pain, and 11 had a 50 percent reduction in pain. If treatment such as physiotherapy, chiropractic therapy and exercises have not helped your symptoms, then saline injections may offer relief.

A disc prolapse in the lower back can irritate a nerve and cause sharp shooting

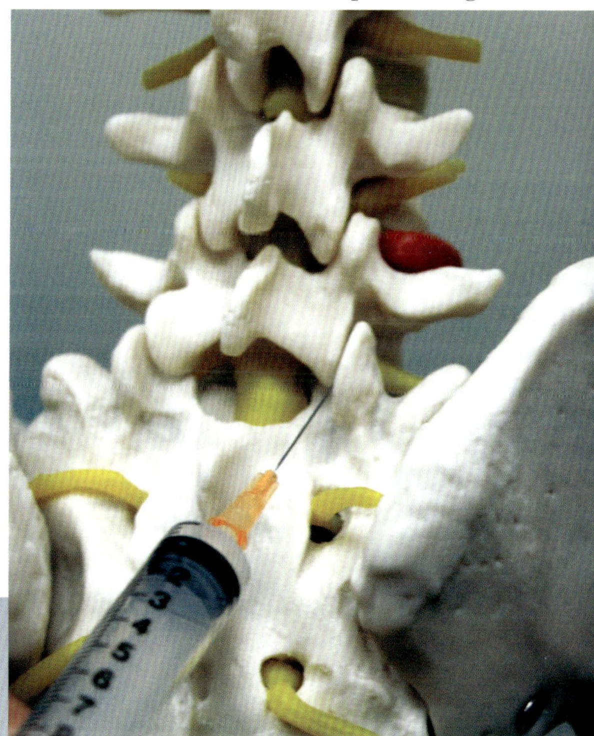

Figure 6.5
Injection of the facet joint.

pain, pins and needles and numbness in the leg. Steroids can be injected around the nerve to improve these symptoms.

The facet joints may also be injected with steroids under X-ray or ultrasound (*Figure 6.4*). Another treatment for the facet joints is to destroy the nerves that supply the joint, therefore stopping any electricity conducting pain to the brain. The nerve can regrow, but the procedure may provide 12 or more months' relief from pain.

Surgery for lower back pain

Sometimes, lower back pain does not respond to conservative management and surgery is considered. If severe back pain is ruining someone's life and their scan shows a problem amenable to surgery, then the two most common operations are discectomy and fusion. Disc replacement is a more recent surgical development.

Discectomy

Discectomy is the removal of part of the disc that has squeezed out of the disc wall *(Figure 6.5)*. Usually, the disc will shrink with time, but sometimes the disc prolapse is so large that it persists and continues to compress the nerve that supplies the leg. Inversion therapy has been shown to reduce the operation rate in disc prolapse so is worth trying prior to considering discectomy. Return to work after a discectomy often depends on the type of job that the person does, with quicker return to work for desk-bound workers than those who perform heavy manual work.

The operation takes approximately one hour, and patients are out of bed and often walking to the toilet on the day of their surgery. Patients usually return home within a few days. Complications can include a recurrent disc protrusion where some more material squeezes out of the disc. This occurs in two to three percent of people in the first year, and in up to ten percent of people in the first ten years after surgery.

Figure 6.5
Discectomy is where disc material is removed from the disc prolapse.

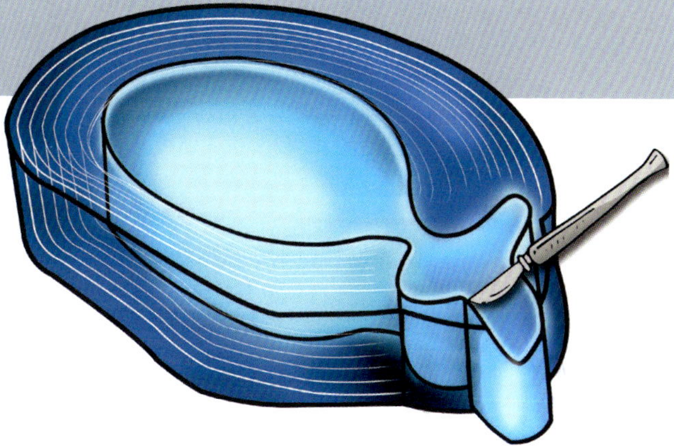

Fusion

In patients where the disc has narrowed and lost the ability to absorb pressure, a fusion can be performed. This is where the bones are fixed together with screws *(Figure 6.6)*, plates or even a cage so that they move as one unit and pressure is alleviated from the disc. A few days' bed rest is required after the operation, but patients usually go home within a week. Walking is the most appropriate exercise immediately after a fusion. After a few weeks, a patient can go swimming. One percent of patients can get post-operative infections, and in up to five percent of patients the vertebrae do not fuse.

In a healthy spine, all the discs absorb some pressure and allow some movement. However, if one level is fused, it can no longer absorb pressure and extra movement and pressure can occur in the discs surrounding the fusion. This can eventually lead to damage of surrounding discs, which may require further levels in the spine to be surgically fused.

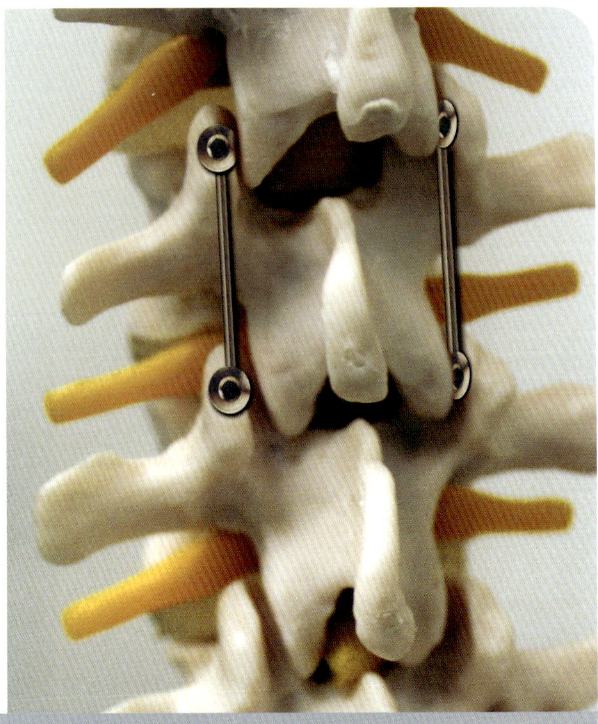

Figure 6.6
A fusion of the lower back.

Disc replacement

Disc replacement has been developed as an alternative to spinal fusion. The damaged disc is replaced with an artificial disc, which is designed to allow some movement in the spinal segment rather than stop movement altogether. This relatively new procedure has been used in Europe for more than 15 years and has recently been approved in the United States. It is still considered experimental compared with spinal fusion. *Figure 6.7* shows a disc replacement between two vertebrae. It is prudent to exhaust all conservative measures prior to considering disc replacement as it is a relatively new procedure and long-term results are uncertain.

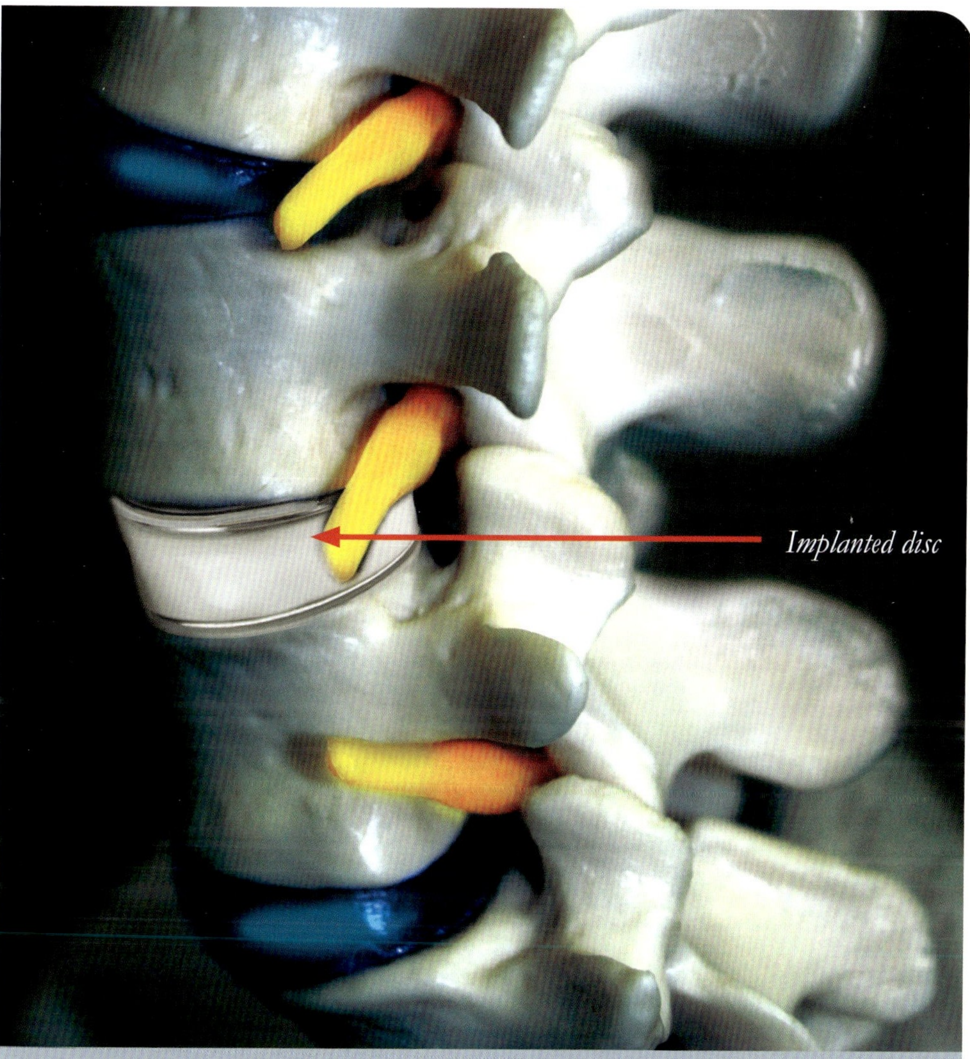

Figure 6.7
A disc replacement showing the metal edges and plastic centre of the implanted disc.

7 CHRONIC LOWER BACK PAIN

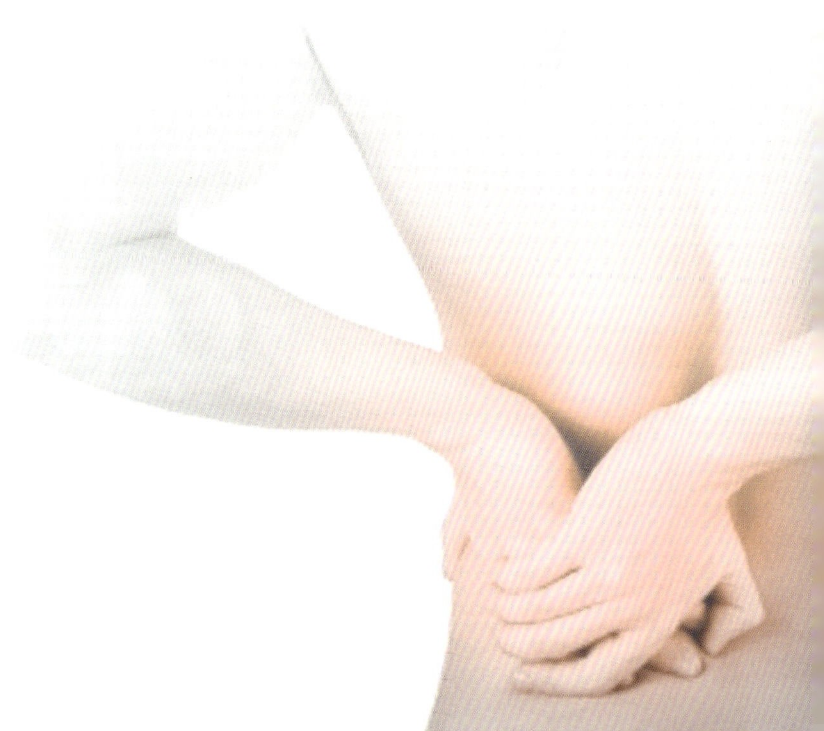

Fortunately, most people with lower back pain improve and return to their normal activities. Around five percent however continue to experience back pain on a daily basis and become limited in their activities. After many years of observing chronic pain patients, I have noticed that living with pain often leads to stress-related conditions such as insomnia, anxiety and depression. Moreover, the risk increases with the number of episodes of back pain experienced. So why do people with long-term pain develop stress-related symptoms? I decided to investigate this question as part of my PhD[8]. I hoped that understanding how these problems develop could lead to solutions for them.

The answer lies in stress chemicals that are released when a patient experiences pain. Adrenaline is the major stress chemical released, and I called the development of these symptoms the Adrenaline Nightmare. Cold, psychological stress, hunger, excess alcohol, poor sleep and viral illness along with pain, can all activate the stress pathways, release adrenaline and perpetuate the Adrenaline Nightmare. Other stress chemicals released in the brain and spinal cord include histamine, serotonin and noradrenaline.

These stress chemicals attach to the brain pain switch increasing electricity and amplifying pain. Furthermore, the stress associated with not being able to work, dealing with insurance companies for compensation, relationship difficulties and loss of self esteem, can add to the release of stress chemicals and perpetuate pain. Life events such as bereavement and separation also increase stress chemicals.

Excess alcohol activates the stress nervous system and leads to the release of stress chemicals. Overnight, the body releases adrenaline which increases the

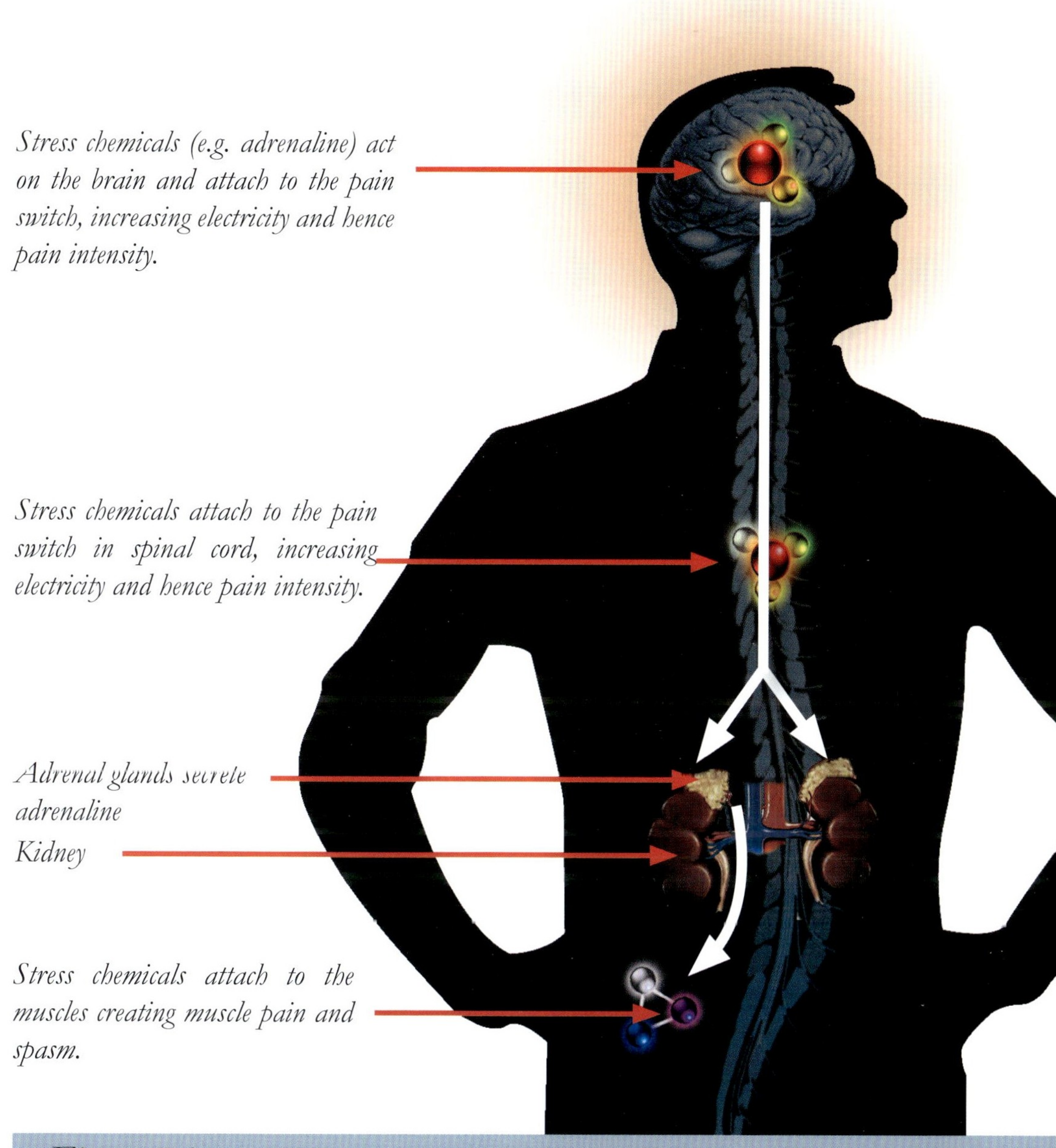

Figure 7.1
Stress chemicals act in the brain and body leading to increased pain and muscle spasm.

electricity in the pain switches in the brain, causing you to wake with headache or even whole body ache in the morning. People often attribute hangover headache to dehydration, but this is unlikely as people in Africa, a part of the world where dehydration is prevalent, suffer very few headaches. Drinking water does however help hangover headache as you flush the adrenaline out of the bloodstream by increasing the urinary excretion of adrenaline.

The release of stress chemicals activates the "fight/flight" response in the body, a very primitive response designed primarily to escape danger. Stress chemicals prepare the body for vigorous physical activity and are depleted by running or fighting. Unfortunately, when released by pain or stress, stress chemicals are not consumed and build up in the brain. Stress chemicals can keep you alert, awake, on edge and anxious. This feeling can disturb sleep and cause you to wake at night due to the smallest disturbance. If stress chemicals continue to build up in the brain, you can even develop panic attacks or depression.

Adrenaline increases blood flow to the muscles up to ten-fold for running and fighting, sharpens the eyesight and hearing, and reduces blood flow to all the non-emergency organs in the body. To supply the muscles with increased blood flow, the heart must pump vigorously, often resulting in palpitations (an awareness of heart beat) and increased blood pressure.

Adrenaline reduces blood flow to the skin and switches off skin repair cells, leading to dry skin. Blood flow is reduced to the hands and feet causing cold hands and feet (often called Raynauds phenomena), which is a sign of an overactive stress nervous system.

The digestive system is not essential when faced with a life threatening situation, and adrenaline release can lead to a 40 percent reduction in blood flow to the gut. Digestive enzymes and movement of the gut are also reduced, leading to irritable bowel syndrome. Stress also leads to the development of stomach ulcers.

Glucose and fats are released to provide fuel for the vigorous physical activity required while escaping danger. However, when adrenaline is released for pain, glucose or fat is not consumed by vigorous physical activity and can aggravate diabetes and heart disease. Furthermore, stress chemicals constrict the blood vessels of the body and increase blood pressure. The combination of raised glucose and fats in the blood stream with increased blood pressure, is the reason stress is the major cause of heart disease worldwide.

Depleting stress chemicals

When treating patients with long-term pain it is essential to advise patients how to manage the stress response. Managing the factors that increase stress chemicals such as excess alcohol, poor sleep, psychological stressors and reducing pain are essential in achieving a long-term successful result. Adding therapy that reduces stress chemicals such as heat, exercise and relaxation helps reduce pain and stress-related conditions. The body has also evolved to release lower levels of stress chemicals when we age. This results in people over 65 years-old often having a calmer disposition and an improvement in certain pain conditions such as headache and migraine.

How can you prevent the build-up of stress chemicals? Reducing stress chemicals in the circulation will help the distress and insomnia that patients often develop from chronic pain. Stress chemicals can either be consumed or their production can be reduced.

Regular exercise improves blood flow throughout the body and will deplete stress chemicals. I recommend that patients exercise for 30 minutes at least four times a week to help them return to a normal life. Exercise can be performed in two bursts of 15 minutes if fatigue is a problem.

Heat reduces the activity of the stress nervous system. Normally, the activation of the stress nervous system constricts the blood vessels in the skin, but heat causes these blood vessels to dilate. When the skin's blood vessels dilate, a signal is sent to the brain to tell it to stop producing stress chemicals

CASE STUDY: *Tania*

When *Tania* was 14 years-old she was practising gymnastics and developed right knee pain that continued, despite two operations. By the time I reviewed her at the age of 28, her pain had spread into the lower back, mid back, neck and arms. She also experienced headache and migraine frequently. Her sleep was disturbed and she felt tired all the time. Tania was also depressed and her weight had doubled over the intervening 14 years.

Tania had difficulty performing housework and often took codeine before washing dishes to manage her pain. She had also started taking several other medications including naproxen, codeine, amitriptyline, omeprazole and citalopram, as well as multiple vitamin supplements.

I advised Tania about the effects of the stress nervous system and how it can spread pain. She was given saline injections into the lower back muscles and ligaments. She started aquajogging and attending the sauna three to four times a week to burn off adrenaline and improve her fitness.

I reviewed Tania two weeks later. Not only had she noticed a reduction in pain, but she had reduced her codeine, naproxen and amitriptyline intake. After one month, Tania had stopped all her medications. She was starting to sleep well, had increased energy and her mood had improved. Her migraines also subsided, and her pain was now limited to her left knee.The muscles around the knee were treated and she was given exercises to help the alignment of her kneecap. She was discharged, approximately three months after her first appointment.

After her pain settled, Tania continued to exercise and lost a significant amount of weight, dropping from a size 24 to size 16. She also noticed an increase in energy. I recently received an email from Tania stating she was in good health and had completed the local around the bays fun run.

such as adrenaline. The deep relaxation felt after a sauna is due to this reduction in the activity of the stress nervous system.

A clinical trial, performed as part of my PhD, on people suffering daily headache, showed severity and duration of headache reduced on average over 40 percent after they attended the sauna for 20 minutes three times a week for six weeks. The improvements were sustained a year after the trial finished. If you can tolerate heat, then this is an excellent way to reset your stress pathways that does not require medication. If you cannot stand the heat for long, then after five to ten minutes leave the sauna, have a warm shower then reduce the temperature to cold. This will reset your temperature switch and allow you to get back in the sauna. Remember to drink plenty of water. Other options include hot baths and spa pools, although these do not provide the same intense heat as a sauna.

Breathing exercises also work in the same way as heat by signalling the stress nervous system to relax. Instead of breathing by expanding the chest you need to learn to breathe by moving the abdominal muscles. This results in deeper and slower breaths which reduce the activity of the stress nervous system.

Deep relaxation or meditation reduces the activity of the stress nervous system and subsequent production of stress chemicals. In one large study[9], 20 minutes of meditation per day helped reduce headaches by 95 percent. Any relaxation therapy may help if performed 20 minutes daily, although meditation seems to have the most supporting evidence.

Sleep disturbance and fatigue

Sleep disturbance creates fatigue by upsetting the pattern of cortisol release. Cortisol is another chemical released during stress. It also has a daily release pattern that is important in maintaining energy. Cortisol levels can be thought of as an indicator of your battery charge with high levels in the morning (giving rise to feeling like a "box of birds") and low levels in the evening, leading to tiredness. Cortisol increases overnight with a slow, steady rise in the first six hours of sleep, followed by a rapid rise in the last few hours of sleep *(Figure 7.2)*. When you wake,

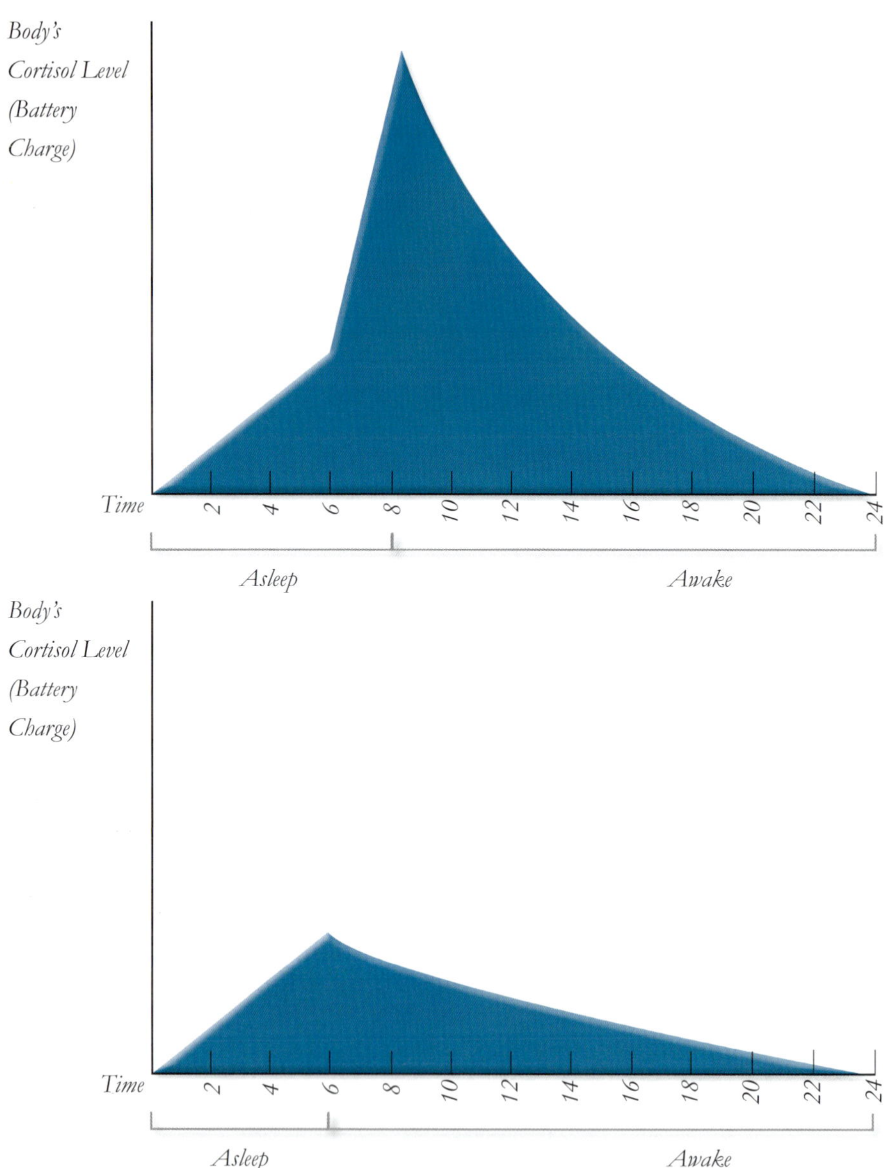

Figure 7.2

The top graph shows the normal patterns of cortisol secretion. The highest levels are present in the morning and give you energy. If you sleep less than four to six hours, you may wake without the cortisol levels reaching their peak, as shown in the second graph.

the battery charge is maximum. If you wake before you have slept for six hours, your levels of cortisol are likely to be sub-optimal and you will feel tired. Over many months of poor sleep, the production of cortisol loses its pattern and, after several years, the level of cortisol is often depleted as the gland suffers burnout (often called adrenal fatigue).

The pattern of cortisol release can be best understood by looking at jetlag. Jetlag is due to a mismatch between your cortisol levels and your time zone. If you travel halfway around the world your battery will be fully charged at night instead of in the morning. You feel energy at night and are tired in the morning. Over a week or so you adjust to your new time zone as your cortisol levels change.

Sometimes it is difficult to restore a sleep pattern. Medications may be useful in the short term by helping to restore a sleep pattern which leads to improved energy and allows you to exercise. If you are taking sleeping tablets such as diazepam, temazepam or zopiclone, then it is wise to take these no more than three times a week. If taken every day, they stop working as the brain gets used to the tablet and addiction can occur. Other sedatives including amitriptyline, Tegretol and quetiapine belong to a range of tablets that are used for epilepsy, depression and psychosis. One of the main benefits of these tablets is that they all cause sleepiness, as they act on receptors that cause sedation. These can be taken daily. Trial and error will determine which suits you best and causes the fewest side effects. Some people may be intolerant to certain medications. If you cannot tolerate one tablet, try another until you find one that suits you. Tablets can be a useful addition to more natural remedies such as going to a sauna, especially in the short-term to improve sleep.

In patients with chronic sleep deprivation and fatigue where the adrenal gland has stopped producing cortisol (adrenal fatigue), fortunately the gland has the ability to restore its normal pattern of cortisol production and hence restore energy. Sleeping well for seven to eight hours per night for several months is required for the function of the adrenal gland to start functioning again and let us wake feeling refreshed. Ensuring minimal sleep disturbance from noise, avoiding caffeine drinks, stimulating activity late at night, regular exercise, sauna and relaxation as well as medication may all combine to improve sleep.

Conclusion

Lower back pain is often difficult to understand by those who do not suffer from it. There are no visible signs such as a plaster cast or deformity for your suffering; it is essentially invisible. Often patients do not mention their problem to others, including health professionals, due to the lack of empathy and solutions.

For the health professional who treats lower back pain it is best to give advice on disc pain as this is the most common source of lower back pain: information on the structure and function of the disc, postures to reduce disc pressure and avoiding activities or postures that increase disc pressure. Tablets can be prescribed to help reduce pain and to help sleep if sleep is disturbed. Patients appreciate finding out the cause of their lower back pain and management strategies aimed at the cause of symptoms. If a patient's pain does not subside or recurs frequently, it is essential to find the cause of their symptoms in order to understand how to deal with their symptoms. An X-ray may help if lower back pain has been present many years, otherwise an MRI scan is the best test to show the disc structure. Tests must be correlated with the pain story and examination findings to ensure what is found on the tests correlates with the symptoms. Once the patient knows what is causing their pain, they can adopt activities/postures that will lessen pain and discard activities/postures that aggravate their pain.

I worked on this book over a three-year period and, during that time, I have tested the management strategies described with hundreds of patients who had suffered from lower back pain. Some patients had been in pain for just a few months, others for over 20 years. Many patients improved substantially by simply using inversion, exercising regularly and changing postures. This has allowed them to reduce dependence on healthcare providers as well as stop taking medications. If you suffer from lower back pain I hope this book helps you understand and manage your pain.

Glossary

aberration Deviation from the normal or expected.

acupuncture Procedure adapted from traditional chinese medicine in which fine needles are placed into the skin and muscles for therapeutic purposes and pain relief.

adrenaline Stress chemical released from the adrenal glands when the body is under stress.

anaesthetic /local anaesthetic Agent injected into an area of the body to numb it or take away sensation.

annular ligament/annulus fibrosis/ring ligament Tough circular ligament surrounding the soft core of an intervertebral disc.

annular tear Tear or hole in the outer disc wall of an intervertbral disc.

bone scan Nuclear scanning test that finds areas of increased bone turnover.

chronic pain Pain lasting for longer than three months.

congenital abnormality/variation Defect or variation present at birth.

CT scan Computed tomography scan where multiple X-rays are taken and used to form a cross-sectional picture of the area.

diagnosis Nature or cause of a disease or injury.

disc Shock absorber (washer) in between the bones of the spine.

discectomy Surgical removal of a herniated or protruding disc.

disc bulge Small protrusion of a disc seen on an MRI scan.

disc prolapse Condition in which the disc no longer sits within its normal confines and the gel centre of the disc squeezes through the ring ligament.

disc replacement Artificial implant used in place of a disc.

electrical therapies Use of electrical energy as a medical treatment.

end plate Surface of the vertebra that comes into contact with the disc.

facet joint/zygoapophyseal joint Synovial joint that helps support the weight of the body and controls movement between individual vertebrae of the spine.

fusion Surgical technique that joins two or more vertebrae together to stop them from moving.

genetic predisposition Having the genes that make a condition more likely to occur.

hard tissues Mineralised tissues like bone and cartilage.

insomnia Difficulty getting to sleep or staying asleep.

invasive treatment Treatment that involves entering the body.

ligament Band of fibrous tissue connecting two bones together.

lumbar spine/lower back Refers to the lowest five segments in the spine.

manipulation Manual therapy which employs thrust techniques to stretch joints.

manual therapy Hands-on treatment, for example: massage, mobilisation and manipulation.

migraine Hereditary predisposition to sensory amplification (light, sound, touch, pain and smell). Most commonly associated with severe headache characterised by sharp pain that usually affects one side of the head. The headache is often accompanied by nausea, vomiting, and visual disturbances.

mobilisation Process intended to make a joint mobile by gentle forces.

MRI scan Magnetic Resonance Imaging produces high quality images of soft tissues such as the disc in the spine using magnetic technology.

musculoskeletal medicine Medicine for both acute and chronic conditions of the musculoskeletal system, i.e. muscle, joints, nerves, ligaments, cartilage and spinal discs.

pain Sensory and emotional experience that creates physical and psychological suffering.

pain pathway Route along which pain signals are sent to the brain.

pain switch Relay switch in the brain or spinal cord that conducts pain.

prolotherapy Injection therapy used to treat various types of chronic pain.

psychiatrist Doctor who specialises in the diagnosis and treatment of mental health disorders.

psychologist Professional who studies the mind and looks at behaviour, cognition and social influences.

receptor Group of nerve endings that responds to stimuli.

referred pain Pain felt at a site other than that where the pain originated.

sacro-iliac joint Joint in the bony pelvis between the sacrum and the ilium of the pelvic girdle, where they meet on either side of the lower back.

saline Salt solution.

side effects Undesirable effect of a drug or therapy.

soft tissues Tissues that connect, support or surround other tissues or organs, and are not made of bone, e.g. muscles, ligaments and tendons.

steroids Group of synthetic hormones that promote the growth and healing of tissue.

stress chemicals Chemicals like adrenaline that are released into the bloodstream when the body is stressed or in pain.

sympathetic nervous system/stress nervous system The nervous system in the body that detects changes (stress), such as heat, cold and psychological stress, causing the release of stress chemicals.

tendon Fibrous tissue that connects muscle to bone.

vertebrae Bony segments that form the spine.

X-rays Electromagnetic radiation that is used to take pictures of the bones in the body.

References

1. Price, C 2005 The management of low back pain. In Holdcroft, A. & Jaggar, S. (ed) Core Topics in Pain 2005 Core Topics in Pain. Cambridge University Press, Cambridge, ch 22: 151- 157.
2. Woolf AD & Pfleger B 2003 Burden of major musculoskeletal conditions. Bulletin of the World Health Organization 81(9): 646-656.
3. Kanji, G. 2005 Convergent referred pain mechanisms: the research and implications for clinical practice. Australasian Musculoskeletal Journal, 2: 124-126.
4. Sheffield FJ 1964 Adaptation of tilt table for lumbar traction. Archives of Physical Medication and Rehabilitation Sept: 469-472.
5. Prasad M, Gregson BA, Hargreaves G, Byrnes T, Winburn P & Mendelow D 2012 Inversion therapy in patients with pure single level lumbar discogenic disease: a pilot randomized trial. Disability & Rehabilitation 34(17): 1473–1480.
6. Kanji, G 2006 The management of lumbar spine pain. Australasian Musculoskeletal Journal, 11(2): 91-97.
7. Yelland, M, Glasziou, P, Bogduk, N, Schluter, P & McKernon, M 2004 Prolotherapy injections, saline injections and exercises for chronic low-back pain: a randomised trial. Spine 29(1): 2126-2133.
8. Kanji, G 2012 The sensory amplification of pain- The adrenaline model of headache causation. PhD thesis in print.
9. Kiran, U, Behari, M, Venugopal, P, Vivehanandhan, S & Pandy, R 2005 The effect of autogenic relaxation on chronic tension headache and in modulating cortisol response. Indian Journal Anesthesia, 49(6): 474-478.

Further reading

An excellent text book written for health professionals is - Bogduk N Clinical Anatomy of the Lumbar Spine and Sacrum. Churchill Livingstone. 3rd edition.

Index

A
acupuncture, 84
adrenaline, 92
anaesthetic, 84
annular ligament, 23
annular tear, 26

B
bone scan, 53

C
chronic pain, 92
congenital abnormality/
variation, 36
CT scan, 53

D
disc, 22
discectomy, 86
disc bulge, 27
disc prolapse, 28
disc replacement, 88

E
electrical therapies, 21
endplate, 25, 29

F
facet joint, 34
fusion, 87

G
genetic predisposition, 10**I**
insomnia, 97
invasive treatment, 4

L
ligament, 21
lumbar spine, 18

M
manipulation, 83
manual therapy, 82
migraine, 10
mobilisation, 82
MRI scan, 51

P
pain, 10
pain pathway, 11
pain switch, 11
prolotherapy, 85
psychiatrist, 1
psychologist, 1

R
receptor, 10
referred pain, 13

S
sacro-iliac joint, 42
saline, 85
side effects, 79
soft tissues, 19, 21
steroids, 86
stress chemicals, 94
sympathetic nervous system/stress nervous system, 92

T
tendon, 21

V
vertebrae, 23

X
X-rays, 49

Acknowledgements
Thanks to everyone who helped in shaping this book. Preehya Patel who designed the cover, all the illustrations and layout. Annemaree Naylor, Pamela Rivers and Janene Bone who read the book and provided valuable feedback. Thanks to Associate Professor Rachel Page for editing the book and Kylie Sutcliffe who went over the many versions of the manuscript. Thanks to Mary Varnham for her thoughtful input. Thanks goes to all the patients who were instrumental in helping me understand pain and gain insights that have lead to the writing of this book. Finally, my love and appreciation goes out to my wife, Sathna and my children Ataya, Keelan and Jessica for reading drafts and their patience and understanding.

Dr Giresh Kanji (Wellington)
May 2013

Second Edition
Thanks to all those who have purchased the book. The valuable feedback has confirmed that it is easy to read and understand. The title has been changed and we have made slight amendments to the text.

Dr Giresh Kanji
November 2013